FUTURE MAN

HOW TO EVOLVE AND THRIVE
IN THE AGE OF TRUMP, MANSPLAINING,
AND #METOO

TIM SAMUELS

Arcade Publishing • New York

First North American Edition

First published in the English language under the title *Who Stole My Spear?* This updated edition published by arrangement with The Random House Group Limited.

Arcade Publishing books may be purchased in bulk at special discounts for sales promotion, corporate gifts, fund-raising, or educational purposes. Special editions can also be created to specifications. For details, contact the Special Sales Department, Arcade Publishing, 307 West 36th Street, 11th Floor, New York, NY 10018 or arcade@skyhorsepublishing.com.

Arcade Publishing® is a registered trademark of Skyhorse Publishing, Inc.®, a Delaware corporation.

Visit our website at www.arcadepub.com.
Visit the author's site at www.tim-samuels.com.

10 9 8 7 6 5 4 3 2 1

Library of Congress Cataloging-in-Publication Data

Names: Samuels, Tim, author.
Title: Future man: how to evolve and thrive in the age of Trump, mansplaining, and #MeToo / Tim Samuels.
Description: First North American edition. | New York: Arcade Publishing, [2019] | Includes bibliographical references.
Identifiers: LCCN 2019006082 (print) | LCCN 2019009482 (ebook) | ISBN 9781628729955 (ebook) | ISBN 9781628729931 (hardcover)
Subjects: LCSH: Men—Humor. | Masculinity—Humor.
Classification: LCC PN6231.M45 (ebook) | LCC PN6231.M45 S26 2019 (print) | DDC 818/.602—dc23
LC record available at https://lccn.loc.gov/2019006082

Cover design by Erin Seaward-Hiatt
Cover illustration: iStockphoto

Printed in the United States of America

Dedicated to:

(Fill in when commitment embraced)

CONTENTS

CONTENTS

PREFACE TO THE AMERICAN EDITION

Even given the unpredictabilities of Washington, DC, it's hard to imagine a Men's March snaking its way through the capital. Hundreds of thousands of regular guys, proudly sporting their self-knitted, baby-blue "Penis hats," trudging up Constitution Avenue to assert their trampled masculinity. Signs defiantly held aloft—WHAT HE SAID, THE MENPIRE STRIKES BACK— by a phalanx of hairy hands.

The plight of the male in the United States today hardly seems like something to take to the streets about. A nation run by a hypermacho president presiding over an 80 percent male Cabinet. Where women's rights over control of their bodies, which had been established for decades, suddenly appear perilously vulnerable. And the #MeToo revelations of grim male abuses of power keep on flowing.

Nope, it's not men's moment. If anything, it feels like a time of male reckoning.

Yet, paradoxically, it's now more than ever that we need to understand what's truly going on with men. To move beyond lazy stereotypes and grapple with the messy, nuanced, sometimes contradictory realities of being a man today. Because masculinity is a deeply powerful—and potentially toxic—force in our lives and politics. One that's fueling democracy-buggering populism, driving a public health epidemic that's rolling back centuries of progress, and causing spasms of shocking violence.

Men not feeling like men is a geopolitical force to be reckoned with. But good luck saying that in the office and expecting any faces to remain straight; or, to raise the stakes, defending that proposition on a date in New York when you were hoping for a little loving later.

Embattled masculinity is a blasé blind spot that many (fellow) liberals dismiss at their peril. The right in the US, on the other hand, seems to *convey* a more intuitive feeling for men, even if it's just man-whistle politics.

To understand the ascent of Trump (and the wider populist surges around the world), you need to delve into the souls of some men, into what's keeping men awake at night.

Perhaps the best way to understand how masculinity can have such socio-political potency is through one particular prism: loss.

Witness poker players on a losing streak: the heedless bets and reckless bluffs to desperately recoup their chips. Because loss at the casino doesn't just drive us crazy, it truly hurts. Psychologists say the sensation of *losing* something has twice the intensity of any pleasure we might accrue. Losing keeps you awake at night. It fuels rage and regret. The desperation to win back what we've lost is what truly makes us lose our heads.

And after two hundred thousand years of having one heck of a *Homo sapiens* hand, some men have now hit a serious losing streak.

THE FLOP IN NORTH CAROLINA

I've had the true pleasure—except when I was obliged to dress up as a giant latex sperm—of spending much of the last two years crisscrossing the United States while reporting for National Geographic TV and the BBC. Along the way, when not being blown out by Bernie Sanders or bemoaning our dwindling sperm counts (separate stories, I should note), I've had a chance to see male power in its pomp in Washington, DC, and Wall Street yet also come face-to-face with those messy manly realities— and that fug of loss.

In the foothills of the Appalachians in North Carolina, the tiny town of North Wilkesboro must once have oozed masculinity. During Prohibition, stock-car racing evolved in these mountainous parts as a way for moonshiners to outrun law enforcement in customized cars (engines souped-up, back seats removed to squeeze in more liquor). This bootlegging by-product morphed into the sporting behemoth of NASCAR racing, and North Wilkesboro, population four thousand, had its very own top-level racing track. The town punched beyond its sporting weight too.

"This was a factory town. We had the biggest furniture factories, biggest textile factories, in the United States," local lawyer Mike Cooper tells me. We're standing in front of the NASCAR speedway. The paint is peeling, the gates shuttered, and a couple of dogs loll around. The track closed in the mid-nineties.

"This was the focal point of a culture and then it got taken away from folks. For rural Southerners, it's the NFL, it's a matter of pride."

Needless to say, the furniture and textile factories are also shuttered. "When you're a young guy and you're working-class and you lose that, you go from being the pride of society to not having a place, not knowing what your identity is," Cooper says.

The crumbling racetrack, the dollar stores that surfaced in the wake of the factory closures, and the chicken processing plant that's now the biggest employer in town are the mere physical manifestations of losses that leach into rural and rust belt America. Into the souls of men.

Tot up the sleep-destroying, angst-generating tally of potential losses to guys that can stem from not having steady, meaningful work. Loss of

income, status, identity, wider belonging, daily purpose, relationships
. . . and health.

With his soft-spoken doctor's demeanor, Haider Warraich, MD, doesn't
seem like the sort of chap to liberally toss around terms like *crisis.* But
once we've dispensed with the pleasantries and green tea in his office at
the Duke University Medical Center in Durham, a two-hour drive east of
North Wilkesboro, after multiple uses of *concerning,* he lands on *crisis.*
And then goes all in on "public health emergency."

That emergency is men's health.

"Starting from, say, the beginning of the nineteenth century, our lifes-
pans—men's and women's—have increased every single year, about three
months every single year. There is no precedent for this in human history," notes the clinical researcher and cardiology fellow.

But, bucking these historical trends, male mortality in the United
States is now starting to go into reverse. Middle-aged men, adrift in this
economy, are actually turning the tide of evolutionary longevity.

"There has been research that shows this inability to participate in the
modern economy is having an effect on increasing rates of premature
deaths, from heart disease, opioids, and suicides in middle-aged men."

An unprecedented historical phenomenon, yet there's barely a public
shrug, let alone an outcry. "It's hard for people at large to feel bad for
men."

Dr. Warraich diagnoses two underlying male-centric conditions behind
this mortality reversal: "increased risk-taking and not enough self-care."

In a Venn diagram of male behavior, sitting within the crossover
between reckless and self-destructive is the opioid epidemic—which is
killing four people a day in North Carolina (twice as many men as
women). Its impact is inescapable. In the liberal city of Asheville, a guy
named John told me he was so out of it he once didn't leave the house for

eight months. Mike, a North Wilkesboro lawyer, revealed that he was addicted in college. Tim, a former logger in the small town of Burnsville who's been clean for ten years, can list on one hand his school friends who are still alive. In his addicted days, he blew the inheritance from his mother on a Corvette and led seventeen police cars on a high-speed chase to the Tennessee border. Moonshine muscle memory.

CHIPS ARE DOWN

Men on their economic downers are primed for something reckless—something radical.

When life has dealt you a bum hand and that agonizing losing streak shows no sign of abating, why, on a purely rational level, would you want the game to go on with the same rules as usual? As a white guy especially, the odds were supposed to be stacked in your favor, but instead you are struggling to make ends meet—so why *not* support a politician who's willing to tip the whole table over, no matter what the consequences or how unpalatable some of his beliefs might be? What have you got to lose?

"Increased risk-taking and not enough self-care"—spreading to the body politic.

And supercharge that economically driven angst with another powerful form of loss: cultural. The sense—whether real or, just as powerful, perceived—that the cultural tides are turning against men. That the scales aren't just being evened out but might be tipping against men. That some men aren't being treated fairly *because* of their gender.

Feeling unable to speak freely, for example, men are preemptively self-censoring and keeping silent, knowing that a misjudged or misconstrued comment can wipe out reputations and jobs (even for seventy-two-year-old Nobel Prize–winning cancer scientist Sir Tim Hunt). Or seeing how due process can wobble—and snap judgments get handed down—when a #MeToo-type allegation is made.

None of this is to *justify*. Nor somehow suggest that the patriarchy wasn't due for a corrective, or that there wasn't vile male behavior in urgent need of comeuppance. It is to try to understand how a vast swath of men has come to feel so vulnerable and defensive: how they've become a time bomb of toxic testosterone, poised for populist touch paper.

Wilkesboro, where NASCAR was eclipsed by chicken processing, lies in Wilkes County. It voted 76.6 percent for Donald Trump. Nationally, Trump picked up 72 percent of the white rural male vote. Five months earlier, my country had voted to leave the European Union, and a majority of men cast their ballots for Brexit. A rightwing nationalist party is now back in the German parliament for the first time since the Nazis; 69 percent of Alternative for Germany's supporters are male.

Of course, the destabilization of the entire Western liberal order can't be reduced to blokes being pissed off. Radicalism draws nourishment from a myriad of roots, like plain old bigotry or the mendacity of politicians.

But as we survey the upheavals taking place around the world, let's not dismiss the impact of depleted masculinity coming home to roost. A pounding on the door—*Hi, honey, we're home*—by men burdened by their losses.

Even if we're not at the hat-knitting stage, let's take men seriously.

* * *

Fear not: what follows isn't an overearnest analysis of gender relations. Rather, it's more the overhonest confessions of an Americanophile Englishman trying to work out what's going on with men these days. One who's still figuring out: how do you not scupper a hot date by saying you've written a book about the plight of men?

FUTURE MAN

FUTURE MAN

1
INTRODUCTION:
WHO STOLE MY SPEAR?

It's the adult equivalent of wetting the bed.

In the vague, vast open-plan office at the BBC, it began as a robust creative exchange with a boss about a documentary that they wanted me to make—and I, self-righteously, considered a flawed concept. (I was, of course, entirely wrong—and to this day people still cite the stratospheric viewing figures the film later attained with a less-stroppy filmmaker.)

Two adults having a forthright exchange over a film. The everyday stuff of which broadcasting is made. The boss's voice began to rise. The tone became more personal (something about *who did I think I was?*); typing across the office dropped to a light, intermittent tapping as the collective decided that this could be a juicy one. The voice rose, the tone changed—and something just shifted inside. As I stood my corner—*this really is a cynical film people will see straight through*—I could detect a catch developing in the back of my throat.

You don't know how lucky you are . . .

A stinging started to form at the back of my eyes. Keyboards silent.

Who the hell do you think you are?

Holy shit.

Are these *tears* forming?

Male tears have no place in the office. In fact, I've never seen a man cry at work. Over the years, I've probably seen half a dozen women run to the loo, friends in tow, returning a few minutes later to sympathetic nods and encouraging smiles; slightly bloodshot but with no damage to their status. Really, no big deal.

But for a man to burst into tears at work and remain unscathed? He might get away with it if he'd just taken a call saying that his entire family (and the dog) had been swallowed by a sinkhole. Or if he'd just been given ten minutes to live by a consultant.

As I willed the tear ducts to desist immediately, the mere prospect of a couple of tears popping out in the middle of the second-floor brainstorming area invoked the same full pants-down shame I had not felt since the summer of 1983 on a Scouts-style trip—when, unable to fathom how to undo the fastenings on a tent during the night, I mortifyingly had to release the contents of my bladder into the sleeping bag while the other boys slept.

But I wasn't an eight-year-old trapped in a tent. I was a journalist who'd worked undercover in Northern Ireland, faced up to fascist skinheads in riots, accused drug dealers in Jamaica of being involved in murder. I was from the gritty north of England and still doing my best to keep that Manchester swagger. I'd been punched in the face twice—by bouncers— and laughed it off. And here I was on the verge of actually crying in front of fifty-plus colleagues who by now had given up any pretense of looking at their screens.

Male tears are not on the office menu. Reckoning that I was probably about one more sentence away from the dam bursting, I reached deep for the inner Mancunian.

Fuck this shit.

And stormed off, with an overexaggerated strut that bordered on the simian—off outside to suck in some testosterone from a bummed cigarette.

To this day, I still shudder at what would have happened had I not pushed the Northern-male ejector button in time. Would it still be whispered about at office parties? That time when Tim removed his own gonads and left them in a neat pile by the brainstorming whiteboard.

CHANGING MAN

As I—still awkwardly—redredge the incident, I wonder if there could have been something in that moment that encapsulates the tightrope-balancing act of being a man these days? Looking at the scene forensically, I'd point out that it was telling that it took place at work—something that has become damagingly overdominant in our sense of worth and identity. That the geography was an open-plan office—itself an unnatural source of emasculation that sends our fight-or-flight hormones haywire. That these days work often takes place in the head with none of the satisfying physicality that comes from doing something that breaks you out in a healthy sweat, having achieved something tangible. I'd look inside the mind to investigate what my general angst was at the time—sleep patterns, relationship (or not) stress, how big the particular gap was between my life expectations and the reality. And, being thorough, I'd chalk an outline around the fact that the boss yelling at me was a woman. On some level, could there have been something particularly emasculating—or emotion-inducing—about being shouted at by a female boss? And if we're warily veering off PC norms to explore a cliché, yes, it was one of those women bosses who out-mans any man in sight.

A trivial incident, which thankfully didn't end in tears, but which speaks of the wider state of modern man. There's no way my dad, who became a teenager during the Second World War, would have ended up biting his lip during a work tiff. I imagine that his father, who served in the Great War, might just have had better things to get upset about too.

But to go back just one generation or two is to venture into an unrecognizable male landscape. My father was born a mere three years after women over twenty-one were given the vote in Britain. His father was alive when women were not allowed to be politicians, lawyers, accountants, or vets. My great-grandfather was born into an era when married women weren't even entitled to have their own possessions. And all of them lived in times when careers were for life, and a man's place at home and in society was solidly fixed. Ten thousand years of total male certainty and dominance since we went all agrarian (apparently, we were quite PC on the gender front when hunter-gathering) have collapsed in a matter of decades.

And rightly so. Along with twenty-four-hour pharmacies, the great leaps in equality around gender, sexuality, and race are some of our proudest achievements. There may have been oodles of male certainty a hundred years ago, but there also happened to be racial segregation in the United States, imprisoned gay men in Australia, and rampant slum housing and boarding-house signs declaring "no coloreds, no West Indians" in England. We've come a long way (though a KKK chapter claiming that black and gay "wizards" may join them isn't quite the desired paragon of parity).[1]

Forgive men if, at times, we are a little unsure of our footing. Not only because of the comparatively sudden shift in gender relations, after 10,000 years of having our feet up in those cozy dominant slippers, but also due to the other breakneck social changes afoot, which affect man and woman alike. The media barrage filling our heads with unattainable expectations. Technological intrusion into every nook of life. Work that demands more of our time and our souls than ever but offers less and less security. Few obvious answers from organized religion. Living longer: marriage and monogamy must have been a completely different kettle of fish when life expectancy was forty-five. And a general bewildering array of choice.

In five mindless minutes of swiping on Tinder, I can view more single women than my great-grandfather would have seen in his entire lifetime in his village. Quite what ten minutes on YouPorn would have done to the sexual satisfaction of the stern-looking sepia man married off to his portly-looking cousin is open to speculation.

Of course, what's not changed during these societal upheavals is us. Men. Our bodies have barely evolved since we were cavemen. The same synapses and hormones fire today as those that were triggered to keep us safe from lions wandering over the savannah. But our bodies now seem way out of kilter with how we live. The hormones that flood our body to warn of that lion heading our way now kick in when a hostile e-mail lands in our in-box—and keep on being released well beyond the point at which they've achieved their goal of heightening our senses. Fight, flight, or reply all.

Have we overevolved? Is this way of living—this advanced capitalist Western life—the best way for man to be? Are we really meant to be going to offices each day, hunching over desks, endlessly chasing higher increments of status and money? To come home to an aspirationally monogamous relationship having successfully navigated the modern minefield of dating and the toxic mind pollutant of porn, all the while filling our heads with so much pointless microinformation from the devices we're plugged into that we never give the brain a moment to dwell on the awkward question of what's it all about or wonder whether we've been a bit too hasty in chucking away those bizarre religious rituals that seemed to have served man perfectly well since he could first start to draw on cave walls?

Have we become Man Zero? A low-testosterone, diet version of who we're meant to be? Or is the latest recipe—for all its flaws—the best yet?

Man Zero is a subtler, less predictable taste compared to previous male incarnations—the newfound sensitivity of late eighties/nineties' New Man (*Three Men and a Baby*, *Mrs. Doubtfire*) and the vapid sheen of freshly moisturized Metrosexual Man. We've become discerning consumers, shopping around for our ingredients. From female friends and colleagues we've seen some positive traits, and we rather like the look of them. If metrosexuality was once about raiding your girlfriend's cosmetics bag, today it's about raiding her emotional drawers—pilfering the prized capacity to say what's on your mind.

(It's a two-way exchange, of course. To borrow from that other soft drink, stick on a blindfold and take the Pepsi *gender challenge*: who can tell whether any given behavior at home or work today comes from a man or a woman?)

We scrutinize how our fathers lived—their values, what ultimately made them happy or not—and wrestle with what to cherish or chuck out in the way we bring up our own children. We can be far more tolerant, supportive, nonjudgmental than ever before, but there's an underlying restlessness. A dark note, fueled by the gnawing pressure to become the man we thought we were *meant* to be, and on schedule. Bittersweet, capable of greatness and magnanimity—yet prone to rage and radicalism. Repulsed by #MeToo revelations of abuse yet deep-down paranoid that one day an allegation could somehow come knocking. Untethered by the traditional anchors at home/work/beyond, so as free to fall far and deep as to radically reinvent overnight. Tough yet vulnerable. Contradictions as standard.

We are a peculiar concoction. Yet still bottled in that same hunter-gathering body.

Maybe we men are at our best when faced with a fight for survival (an abyss many of our fathers and grandfathers peered into), when dealing with the fundamentals of life, when there are real consequences to our actions, beyond earning a few more dollars to redo the bathroom.

Sure, we might be richer, safer, healthier, and possibly more emotionally sophisticated than ever before, but has today's man lost something in the process?

This isn't a sappy tirade for men's rights. We are the dominant gender and don't have many glass ceilings to push through, though some industries these days are hardly clamoring for white male applicants. But before any women club me over the head with a rolled-up *USA Today*, I'll spell it out myself.

SEVEN REASONS NOT TO WRITE A BOOK ABOUT MEN'S RIGHTS

1. Women aged 25–34 earn 89 cents for every dollar men of the same age group are paid.
2. Women make up only 22 percent of board directors of Fortune 500 companies.
3. An estimated 100–140 million girls and women around the world have undergone genital mutilation.[2]
4. Women make up less than 8 percent of the world's heads of government.
5. In the US, women were not legally defined as "persons" until 1875.[3]
6. In Yemen, a wife must obey her husband and not leave home without his permission.[4]
7. In the UAE, a man has the right to physically discipline his wife if he does not leave physical marks.[5]

I hear—and support—you. There is no zero-sum gender game here. It's a no-brainer that any man should demand that his sisters, female friends, and any other woman has the same freedoms, rights, and opportunities that he has.

As I say, this isn't a call for a male uprising.

When people talk about a men's rights movement—or meninism—it just doesn't sound like a party you'd want to go to. There's something inherently uncool when the dominant group whines about its plight— like whites feeling discriminated against. Deal with it.

If this isn't a plea for men to form a movement and burn their jock-straps en masse, it is a call to recognize that these are challenging times to be a man. Those roles and certainties cemented over millennia have fallen away. The core male values that were applauded through time—heroism, aggression in the face of conflict, and stubborn individuality—are increasingly frowned upon the more civilized we get (though, confusingly, still idealized by Hollywood). Gender lines are shifting and blurring; rites of passage have fallen by the wayside; bringing up boys has become a crapshoot of contradictions; we are self-censoring to not say anything career-imploding by mistake; and it's tough out there to live up to the expectations knocking around in your head.

Sure, men are the undisputed dominant gender—so much so that they can be called an "invisible" gender not worthy of academic study[6]—but there's a big difference between male power across society and the individual experiences of men. To conflate the two, as some are wont to do—what have *men* got to complain about?—is simplistically to miss the point.

Something really has gone pear-shaped for men in particular areas.

NINE AND A BIT REASONS TO WRITE THIS BOOK

1. Men are three and a half times more likely than women to take their own lives. Tragically, other than accidents, suicide is the biggest killer of males between ten and thirty-four years of age.[7]

2. The prison population is 93 percent male, with men receiving longer sentences than women for similar crimes—63 percent more average jail time for men for federal offenses.[8]

3. Boys lag a year behind girls at reading in every industrialized country and are six times more likely to be diagnosed with attention deficit disorder (ADD) than girls.[9]

4. Men receive custody of children in only about 10 percent of divorce cases in the US.[10]
5. Men develop heart disease ten years earlier than women.[11]
6. Sixty percent of the homeless are men.[12]
7. Men are more often victims of violence than women, and one in three men has experienced contact sexual violence, physical violence, and/or stalking by an intimate partner during their lifetime.[13]
8. Twenty-four of the twenty-five lowest ranked professions in the US are heavily male-dominated.[14]
9. Up to 80 percent of couples at some fertility clinics are now requesting girls.[15]

A Bit. Anesh, from the Indian village of Barshitakli, was jailed for a year for having an affair with a shepherd's wife.[16] Under Indian law, a man can be jailed for adultery—whereas a woman can't.

For all of this statistical doom and gloom, and Anesh's incarceration, these can be great times to be a man. There's never been so much freedom to be who you want to be. Hedonistic fixes abound. And yet: it's not straightforward being a man. Nor is it *the end* of man, as some feminists have gleefully proclaimed, to peddle some books. It's just the latest evolution.

But we ignore the "invisible" gender at our peril. When under threat, masculinity has a habit of morphing and resurfacing throughout history. It doesn't go away, but resiliently pops up in different guises, like the pieces in the old arcade game Whac-A-Mole. And it's often not pretty. In the decades before the First World War, when changes at home and work had left men "soft," tellingly there was a surge in celebrating the martial idea, that war could be good for man. Today, beyond the individual examples of male self-destructive behavior—such as drinking, getting kicked out of school, not seeking mental health help—I'd hazard that the rise of IS/ISIS, a terrible toxic fusion of male alienation and a bastardized form of religious extremism, is partly rooted in suppressed masculinity. When a young man swaps his clothing-store street uniform in Portsmouth for military fatigues in Syria, and leaves behind his suburban nine-to-five (and no doubt sexual frustration) to wield a weapon alongside a band of brothers, surely there's an illusion of masculinity being chased here. Across Europe and Latin America, extremist parties are thriving in countries where men have little economic means of proving themselves to be men. Donald Trump surfed a white male wave to the White House. Whether in individual homes or on the world stage, when masculinity is in short supply, there are consequences.

DEFINITELY MANLY

Some fine female writers—from Elizabeth Gilbert to Caitlin Moran—have brilliantly captured what it's like to be a woman today. It might be useful to put a male experience out there, to be totally transparent about what it's like to be a man today, no matter how personal (or at times puerile) that may seem. And see how our innate masculinity can be indulged without causing havoc.

To be honest, it comes with a certain degree of buttock-clenching trepidation. What can be liberating for a woman to write about might be misconstrued as lewd, offensive, or even sexist in the hands of a man.

And, of course, it is *a* male experience, of a straight white Western man. I'm pretty sure I won't be speaking for a Yemeni chap weighing up whether to let his missus out to go shopping unaccompanied or the middle-aged guy in rural Nigeria about to marry a child bride.

But it just feels like there's a need to try to articulate what it's like to be a man. To share with other men—and women—what's going on in our minds, to greater understand ourselves, to widen what men can talk about, to challenge some of the barely one-dimensional media portrayals of men as buffoons incapable of loading a washing machine, and to see what underpins some of those shocking statistics.

To look up from our phones for a minute, question the very norms we've come to take for granted, and ask: "Is this how a man is meant to live?"

To explore how beholden we still are to our animal instincts (can the relative size of our testes to other apes' ever be an excuse for straying?), how we're really supposed to work, find a mate, hold down a relationship, keep sane, go looking for some sort of spiritual fulfillment, bring up kids, handle the explosion of porn, deal with how we look, see if other guys around the world have got any better ideas, and find ways to spend enough man time with our "pack." And, in jargon speak, maybe to change the conversation around men.

So for all the times over the years a girlfriend has asked, "What are you thinking?" only to be met with a monosyllabic shrug, here's the answer. Probably wished they'd never asked now.

2
BECOMING A MAN (IN THE SAFEWAY PARKING LOT)

It used to be easy to know when you'd finally become a man.

If you happened to grow up among the Seteré-Mawé in Brazil, it was a simple matter of sticking your hand in a glove made of bullet ants—and not wincing during the ten minutes of continuous stinging from the most painful ant in the Amazon. Sure, you might spend several days compulsively shaking afterward, but at least you'd know you were a man by the time your paralyzed arm had come back to life. For a Vanuatuan boy, the rite of passage to manhood was a more straightforward circumcision followed by being thrown off a makeshift hundred-foot bungee tower. Your seventh birthday might not be one you'd look forward to if you'd grown up in the Sambia tribe in Papua New Guinea. Instead of a cake and a few presents, you would have received a sharp stick up the nose—till the blood flow became profuse—then fellated the men in the village, to drink up their "male spirit."[1]

I'd say I got off pretty lightly. The ritual among the assimilated South Manchester Jewish tribe in the late 1980s was to force the thirteen-year-old male to learn a portion of incomprehensible Hebrew by heart then sing it out loud in a synagogue packed with women wearing big hats and men talking business—while truly praying the voice didn't actually break just as Noah was getting busy on the ark—then dine on a buffet of smoked fish–based products. The ritual was sanctified by a plethora of Parker fountain pens. For higher-status members of the tribe, a mildly ostentatious disco would be thrown in the evening, to afford the pimply young man an awkward opportunity to see if any of the girls wanted to "go for a walk" and navigate mouths full of orthodontic metal.

But for me this momentous day—cementing my lineage to Abraham, Isaac, and Jacob—culminated not in a newfound sense of manliness but throwing up in some shrubbery in the parking lot of the Safeway in Hale village. A strange start to manhood.

To be fair, though, I spent more of my childhood in Safeways than in synagogue. And while I can't recall a single word of my bar mitzvah portion, I can still visualize the Safeway's shopping basket with total clarity. Sliced brown bread (white was for *other* people), tasteless tomatoes that were guaranteed to turn any school sandwich rank by lunchtime, limp lettuce that could never dream that it might one day be paired with olive oil instead of a dollop of salad dressing, store-brand instant coffee, canned fruit, frozen mini pizzas the size of a CD harboring trace elements of cheese, and a dented can of whatever happened to be on the sale shelf no matter how unlikely it was to ever be consumed. Oh, the uncontained envy of going to friends' houses where there were actual Marks & Spencer* food items in the fridge—I swear I once spotted hummus. Not to mention the confusion of being served an artichoke at a friend's one day: an artichoke, in the late 1980s, in Manchester. So *nouveau quiche*. We might have been light years away from harnessing the chickpea, but no matter: our austerity Safeway diet was idiosyncratically augmented by a) the health food store that did an unparalleled line in meat-free mince that

---

*The upper echelon of British supermarket chains.

willfully resisted any attempt to absorb flavor, and b) whole industrial-size boxes of broken cookies from the local market.

In retrospect, surviving my childhood seems like a minor nutritional miracle. Barren, leafy-green-free years spent subsisting on pounds and pounds of cornerless Custard Creams cookies, during which anything that ended up on the plate was first thrown into a vat of solidified oil that never left the top of the stove and was never changed. I can't directly blame my dad for the deep-fried diet. His duties extended to hapless foraging at Safeway and dealing in the Manchester underworld of crumbled cookies. Manning the vat was a rotund Irish lady whose sole qualification for providing my and my brother's entire teenage nutritional needs was having once run a truck drivers' café with her truck driver Elvis-impersonator husband. Each day, she came, she fried, we coagulated.

Just a few months before my big coming-of-age day, my cardiac prognosis had been looking decidedly healthier. There were proper family meals around a table, bowls of salad, and puddings that didn't come from cans. But the fruit and veg copped it one turbulent day. In the months beforehand, I could detect a rising strain seeping through the house. Lying in bed at night, I could hear the muffled arguments between my dad and stepmom. They became less muffled. I'd turn up my stereo—but there were always gaps between songs. As a twelve-year-old, though, I had no sense that anything tangible was actually going to result from the arguing. It was a nonspecific unpleasantness to be blotted out. So it came as an utter thunderbolt when one day my dad said, "We're leaving. Pack your bags." I kicked my bedroom door in rage but never slept in that room again.

The bags were packed, and a rocky two-and-a-half-year marriage between my dad and stepmom came crashing down. Bruised and confused, my dad, my older brother Mark, and I relocated that night to a two-up two-down terraced house, and I drew the short straw on the camp bed. The inventory for that divorce was pretty costly. I seemed to lose a stepmother I had dared to call "Mum," three older stepbrothers I totally looked up to, Claude the cat, the piano, a nice house in a posher part of Manchester, and several core food groups.

The resilience of youth is remarkable. I remember calling a friend when we got to the terraced house and having a little cry on the phone as I told her my parents were divorcing, but there were no other moments. It almost became a (reduced) family joke: that Dad had made such a mess by marrying someone he'd known for all of six weeks. Two summers before, Mark and I had returned from a long holiday staying with family in New Hampshire, been picked up from the airport, taken straight to some random family's house, bizarrely made to pose for a group photo, asked if we liked them in the car on the way home, and then told, "That's good, as I'm marrying her, and we're moving in there in a few weeks." Six weeks . . . such an uncharacteristically rash, albeit well-intentioned, decision by a man who is happy to wait six months to time the Costco winter jacket sale to perfection.

Sure, it was something of a blow to lose an entire new family and a house that had a bidet and, as a consequence, to have to spend a small future fortune in sympathetically nodding professionals. But at the time, for a thirteen-year-old, it was a golden ticket not to be wasted. *You have just won first prize in a school sympathy contest: please take as much piss as you can possibly get away with.*

And for the aspiring teenage rebel, Manchester in the late 1980s was the dream place to cash in that ticket. The city was the swaggering, cocksure center of the universe—sticking two Northern fingers up to London and anywhere else that thought highly of itself. Where T-shirts proclaimed On the Sixth Day, God Created Manchester and a cartoon cow mouthed Manchester: Cool as Fuck. Football, music, fashion, anything that was important to young men, we owned it. The sound track of homegrown bands coursed through the city's Victorian streets and pregentrified canals. The Smiths, Joy Division, Buzzcocks, New Order, James, Inspiral Carpets, Charlatans, Happy Mondays, Stone Roses, The Fall—all ours. The Hacienda was pumping out house music to the world. Quiffs, baggy jeans, smiley faces—the outward symbols on our inner style. While the city paused weekly to worship at the red and blue altars of the biggest football club in the world and the iconically underperforming coolest club in the land.

There was also an industrious line in menacing violence. But in a city dubbed "Gunchester" by the tabloids, as rival drug gangs from Moss Side and Cheetham Hill fought a bloody turf war on the streets, the scope of rebellion would be somewhat more modest for a thirteen-year-old from a family who bought brown bread and made him publicly recite a portion of the Torah to accrue fountain pens.

Especially when he went to the poshest school in the city, Manchester Grammar—a meritocratic school that took kids regardless of wealth and turned them all into a bunch of stiffs in highly identifiable owl-crested blazers, and which just happened to be on the doorstep of Moss Side and in literal spitting distance of the fearsome school that rock group Oasis went to. Manchester Grammar was churning out the best grades in the country while really teaching pupils how to slip into the roughest accent at the drop of a hat, or—more often on the public bus I took home—the gob of spit aimed at the poor owl.

During those years, I got away lightly and was robbed only twice. One time was somewhat farcical, when my assailants ran away after a nearby dog barked; the other less so—when two young guys pulled a full-length kitchen knife on me and got away with my wallet, seven pounds, and my bus pass.

So you had to know your place in the pecking order when it came to bad-boy late-eighties rebellion. Fueled by divorce and constrained by

16

going to an exclusive school and having once had access to a bidet, I managed the following in my thirteenth year:

1. School tie worn backward with the thin bit at the front, thus ensuring the owls were plaintively left hanging upside down.
2. Smoking dried banana pith, nutmeg, Indian beedi cigarettes, and a sheet of Latin homework.
3. Buying weed from a drug dealer named Sly in a Moss Side project during school lunchtime—in a major upgrade from nutmeg but a downgrade in common sense.
4. Being the first person in my year to touch under-the-bra boob.
5. Using my brother's birth certificate to get a fake Youth Hostel Association card attesting that I was eighteen.
6. Using this ID to get into the International 2 night club to watch The Waltones play a gig, putting tissue in my ears to drown out the bass, having to go to the school nurse the next day when one of the papers wouldn't budge, and seeing my dad called out of work to take me to the Ear, Nose, and Throat hospital to have it fished out.
7. Becoming a militant vegetarian who handed out leaflets outside the McDonald's on Market Street to bemused families; the leaflets featured a photo of a cow that had been shot through the head in an abattoir and asked, "Would you eat meat if it looked like this?"
8. Temporarily dumping my mates to hang around with boys from two years above, thus allowing access to the back seat of the bus, beer in pubs, and the potential of hallowed older boob.

James Dean it wasn't. But among the South Manchester Jewish community, it was a level of teenage insurrection to be feared. After word somehow spread among the moms of Hale Synagogue, during a momentary pause in hat judging, that I was "doing drugs," my friend Rob was told to keep his distance from me. Grades naturally tumbled at school, academia was shunned in favor of the age-old boyish delight of drawing a phallus on someone else's textbook to see what they could creatively turn the cock and balls into (NASA space rocket and boosters was the default option), and I managed to drag my friends Rob and John down enough that we all got summoned to see the middle school master.

As the three of us lined up in his office for a major league bollocking, he asked if any of us had anything to say for ourselves. From nowhere, like a young Charlie unwrapping a Wonka bar, I caught a glimpse of my golden ticket.

Sir, it's been really hard since my parents got divorced.

Rob saw a lifeline flash before him.

Me too, sir. Mine got divorced too.

Yeah, but that was eight years earlier and he now had the most lavish home any of us had ever seen. A technical pass.

Poor John had nowhere to go. His parents were the epitome of marital stability.

Um, sir, you know, it's been um, it's not always great . . . sometimes . . . uh . . . lately. Sir.

Luckily, it seems my ticket was a group one, and we were all sent back to class rather than home for a couple of ignominious weeks. John's parents remained blissfully married for forty-nine years. The rebellion faded, and even the owl reverted to the right way up.

I look back on those times at school with an almost painful nostalgia. The sheer exhilaration of being around your closest friends, day in, day out. A constant maelstrom of genial mockery. Bestowing simple yet physically literal nicknames: Goofy Deaf Twat, Forest Forehead, Egghead—and Tribal Warfare for the friend who was one day deemed to have three testes despite a lack of supporting evidence.

A blizzard of powdered candy fights, jostling in airless bus lines, ducking from sprays of ink and hot tea, sucker punches, football (you say *soccer*) arguments, industrial-strength wedgies, and aggressively nudging anyone who deigned to talk to a girl. Should a nudge not do the trick, repeated kicks to the back of the knee normally saw off any chance of getting lucky with a girl.

The mocking was merciless, but never caustic. Fooling around was the glue that bonded a brotherhood together. Airtight friendships—underpinned by a real affection and supportiveness—that bordered on the familial. And for me, at the time, I'd take familial wherever I could get it.

I had my dad, my brother, and my surrogate family of rock-solid buddies. And they'd all be at my bar mitzvah party, unlike me.

There was no toxicology test carried out in Safeway's parking lot. I suspect my body was reacting to a vitamin in the buffet it had never encountered before.

The morning had passed without event. I'd spent weeks after school learning my portion of the Old Testament by heart. When my time came, the heavily bearded, barrel-chested rabbi called me up before the congregation. The Smiths T-shirt and cardigan had been swapped for a navy blazer and beige chinos, the Doc Martens replaced by brown brogues. A thirteen-year-old with John Lennon glasses, spiky hair, voice teetering on an octave change, just two months and twenty-two days away from his first bra strap—and now being declared a man in front of his community.

Passing the threshold of manhood didn't feel monumental at the time. But seminal childhood events rarely do as they are occurring. The obsession at the time was less about the coming of age and more about the coming of coming. The kudos that were gained from being able to come were immeasurable. You could see the swagger of the hairy-balled classmates swanning around the changing rooms. I was desperate to join this club by the time I was thirteen. Willing the testes into action, I'd stare down the urethra for any sign of upcoming life, like peering for a distant headlight of an approaching subway. Alas, trains never ran on time in the eighties.

So I sang some Hebrew before the community, was blessed onstage by a rabbi and given some presents, had a medium-size buffet, and missed a small party. Hardly the stuff of knee-trembling anthropology. Yet this was a rite of passage that has endured unbroken for several thousand years. Since the days of desert-wandering, through every historical twist and turn, young males in my "tribe" have experienced a Saturday when the community came together and declared them to be a man. No matter how irreligious I may be, there's something powerful about that lineage. Something that adds extra ballast to being a random organism floating around a spinning planet. I guess at the time I may have taken subliminal succor from the message that *Hey, you might be struggling with a lost sense of nuclear family but here's a wider community you're part of.* Who knows what resonates with the young psyche, but I suspect it can't have harmed to keep me on the straight and narrow.

DO THE RITE THING

Who knows how crucial it is to a healthy male psyche to mark that transition from boyhood to manhood. Fellating village elders might be a step too far, but maybe we have lost something intangible yet important in no longer celebrating a boy's passage to becoming a man. In our rush to become a rational secular society, there's no space for idiosyncratic rituals. Yet for so many cultures, it has been deemed an essential part of a boy's development—often involving elaborate ceremonies to emphasize the responsibilities and values expected of a nascent man and stressing his relationship to the older males in the group.

The Lakota Sioux young man would traditionally fast alone on a bluff or mountaintop until he saw a vision that would become a spiritual guardian for the rest of his life.[2] The twelve-year-old Hopi boy would have been taken to spend six weeks in an area with the older men and then kept from his mother for a year and a half.[3] The young male Nilotic, from the seminomadic cattle herders around the Nile Valley, was taken to the elders' area and allowed to consume the *ghamunga* sacred honey mead. His "birth" to adulthood was further symbolized by his wearing women's skirts and jewelry while eating and acting like a pregnant woman.[4] Whereas getting the seventeenth-century English boy *out* of a skirt and into breeches was seen as the first step to adulthood, with sizable chunks of a family's income spent on the big breeching ceremony.[5]

Colorful, bizarre, and at times borderline brutal, yes—but rites of passage have been shown to have a positive psychological impact. AIDS orphans in Botswana displayed improved mental health and social integration after being taken into the wilderness for sixteen-day rituals that mimicked that country's traditional coming-of-age ceremonies.[6] "Despite the absence of any established initiation rite, young men need one," author Mark Gerzon lamented of American youth back in 1982. Young men need to prove their manhood, he said, and without any rites available to them all they have is violence (a pale imitation of war), sexual conquest, and generally going out of their way to demonstrate that they are in no way feminine.[7]

What rites are available to young men these days? Maybe some form of hazing (if not just plain bullying) in the military and fraternities. Losing your virginity at the earliest available opportunity. And getting a driver's license, occasionally followed within months by wrapping the car around a tree while showing off. Unless you happen to cling to some sort of religious identity, that's probably about it for most in the Western mainstream. For others, it might be sending the first paycheck to the family you've left back home or even committing sexual assault to mark initiation into a gang.[8]

In the decade after Gerzon decried the lack of rites to mark manhood, the rate of murder committed by US teens, aged fourteen to seventeen, increased by 172 percent. Gun killings by juveniles quadrupled. And this explosion of violence was all among young men.[9] Of course, it's not to say that if only there'd been a Western version of the sacred honey or agonizing ant glove, then some kid wouldn't have taken a semiautomatic into school or shot up the local liquor store. Role models, family, education, economic opportunity, and mental health all have huge bearing (which we'll explore).

But it's all set against the wider problem of society not catering to the particular needs that boys and men have. Not marking the transition to manhood is one of the missing pieces in this wider jigsaw. After all, there does seem to be a universal male urge for boys to prove themselves as they become men, whether they live in a wooden hut on a nomadic plain or an Ivy League frat house. And that Whac-A-Mole masculinity ensures that some boys will prove their manhood by whatever means is available—and if violence and getting laid are all that's in reach, so be it.

By not taking a moment to mark when boys become men and harness their innate urges rather than letting them just drift into manhood, we are missing a trick. Not least for the huge number of boys growing up in fatherless homes—more than seven million in the US.[10] Some groups are getting smart about this. Boys to Men runs adventure-based weekends in parts of the United States and beyond for boys to choose the man they want to become—citing the words of the African American abolitionist and social reformer Frederick Douglass, "It is easier to build strong children than to repair broken men." They claim school discipline incidents among attendees decline by 85 percent. A Band of Brothers, based in

Brighton, on the south coast of England, says there's an 80 percent reduction in reoffending among the young men who go through their initiation Quest weekend and mentoring programs.[11] Pathways, in Australia, takes thirteen- to fifteen-year-old boys and their fathers or a male mentor into bush camps for five days.

But these sorts of programs are often geared to at-risk boys. Why can't there be a rite of passage that all boys go through? To drift into tree-hugging fantasy land, wouldn't it be something for the school curriculum to schedule a "becoming a man" camp? In which teenage boys go away for the weekend to lodges with the older males in their extended family (and/or male role models), get busy on the camping and fire-making front, carry out some physical challenges, and hear candid stories and wisdom about relationships and life from the elders, all culminating in some moving moment around the fire. Just to take a beat out of the mania of life to say, *Now you're a man.*

Thanks for the pens, though.

3
THE $3,000 PULLING SCHOOL

HOW TO PICK UP WOMEN
(AND GET BANNED FROM COUNTRIES)

And thanks for the girls too.

Well, at least thanks for herding me into the same space as girls—a dance floor and the cruel whiff of arbitrary rejection—courtesy of the odd bar mitzvah disco. Nonetheless, it was a huge competitive advantage at an all-boys' school, where most fellow pupils were still collecting football stickers rather than life lessons in how to kiss a girl whose mouth is a Venus flytrap of steel and elastic bands. All necessary coursework to master for high school diploma dating, which hopefully then graduates into some degree of relationship proficiency as adulthood kicks in.

So it's bizarre, to say the least, to recently find myself in Miami, in a room of 150 grown men earnestly taking notes in exercise books, jotting down the words of the teacher at the front, who is instructing them how to pull women. What has it come to that men are paying serious money to learn how to talk to women? Is this a prime case study of Man Zero in his castrated habitat?

"Why on earth would you need an excuse to talk to a girl?" the teacher thunders from the front of the room. Scores of baseball caps nod, pencils scribble. There's no type to the guys present, apart from their ages, roughly twenties to forties. White, black, Latino, preppy, sports-shirted, caps forward, caps back, handsome, geeky, menacing GI types—they are all here. And each hanging on every word.

"You'll hear that. 'What is an excuse to approach a girl?' Why the fuck do you need an excuse? The excuse is you're a man, she's a girl [*mimics finger-into-hole action*]. Isn't that enough? You don't need a fucking excuse."[1]

The messiah delivering salvation from emasculation is Julien Blanc, one of the most renowned pickup artists in the business. The guys sitting in a nondescript hotel conference room in the basement of one of the plainer hotels in Miami have traveled from across the United States for the weekend boot camp. Some have driven for days. They have paid up to $3,000 to be here for the course run by Real Social Dynamics. They've watched the videos and read the books, and now they have a chance to rub shoulders with the likes of Julien and Tyler, a small, receding, introspective ginger-haired guy who has defied visual stereotype to become a master at this game. The pickup artists are afforded near rock-star status. A line forms to have photos taken with Julien.

"I don't know what to say. But, like, you're awesome." A young man in his early twenties has reached the front of the line. "You're actually my idol. You've changed my life, to be honest."

He beams, poses for a photo, and slips away to sit back down with his sheepish, somewhat older girlfriend, whom he's brought along so she can see how he was transformed into someone who was able to get together with her. What on earth are these gurus teaching that's so life-changing, that inspires such a following?

The boot camp is a mixture of pop psychology to slap the male ego back into life, with a near-militaristic series of tactics designed for approaching women with maximum chance of mission success. The pop psychology strikes a chord. Why *are* so many men afraid to go up and talk to a woman they like the look of? Why is it only the same overconfident cheeseballs who can just march on over while the rest of us promise ourselves that we will after just one more drink? It's all symptomatic, the gurus argue, that man has lost his way—that we feel like we need permission to be men again.

"Attraction has always been the same. What attracted a cavewoman back in the day is still what attracts a woman today. Is he going to help me survive? Is he going to help me reproduce? Yes or no?" declaims Julien. The crowd murmurs.

To tap into our inner cavemen, the pickup artists espouse a series of behavioral tactics, designed to short-circuit into what today's Wilmas and Betties are innately looking for.

"You don't need to be model-looking to pick up a girl or to make a girl attracted to you. They're not looking at that. They're looking at the behavioral clues, not the visual clues."

Some behavioral clues to supposedly make you more attractive:

- Don't amble apologetically up to a woman; walk over with confidence, but approach in more of a crab-like arc than marching up directly, which can be a bit confrontational.
- Don't be cowed by whoever she is—playfully tease her over something.
- Try to take the woman away from her group to talk somewhere quiet, thus exerting your dominance by separating her from the pack.
- Establish some form of physical contact.
- Attempt to bring other women into the conversation too, thus demonstrating that you have wider social appeal and status.

- Don't overstay your welcome—get out before your banter wears thin.
- Project that you are at the center of your own great party, and it's a party she'll want to be at.

Some of it definitely makes sense. If I think back to moments when I've been on my supposed A game, it's normally when circumstances have conspired to produce some of these conditions: out with mates looking vaguely popular, not trying too hard, naturally being a bit teasing. The pickup artists would argue that, like any other skill, this can be honed and deployed whatever the circumstances. Even sober. Just as you can become a better golfer or poker player, so you can become a more proficient puller—to the point where no woman should be beyond your reach. Just check out Tyler's track record and look at *him*. It's intoxicating stuff. The pencils haven't paused for breath.

For men who have spent their lifetimes standing on the side of the dance floor watching the cocky douchebags swan over to the girls they like, this is manna from heaven. A revolutionary thought: they don't have to be *that* guy anymore. Which is maybe what the young guy whose life had been changed meant. Viewed this way, it is almost a form of cognitive behavioral therapy (CBT). "What's the worst that can happen?" a CBT shrink will often say. So what is the worst that can happen when you pluck up the confidence to go and talk to a girl? Even if you do crash and burn, you tend to feel energized by having at least gone over to give it a try rather than succumbing to the what-ifs. And Julien et al. would say that by repeatedly approaching women, you are normalizing the experience. It will become less daunting with each attempt.

If this were just a room full of shy guys whose lives have been blighted by a lack of confidence in approaching women, it would be an entirely laudable endeavor. But talking to some of the other guys at the camp, you get a sense it's not just for the shy and retiring. One tells me this is his fourth time at camp, his pulling rates have already improved by "six times, bro," and he's come back again because, "I dunno—just hungry." His buddy in a polo shirt nods along with a little too much GI operational seriousness for my liking: "Absolutely."

Another—young, handsome, in a biker jacket—grins ear to ear at the results he's seen from a previous course. "I actually pulled a stripper a few months ago. So that's like, wow, that's huge for me."

This isn't emasculated man. This is modern man as a canny, entitled consumer. He wants the best job, clothes, house, car, holidays, and he believes that with enough effort and expenditure he can get them. So why not apply this to sex? Why not chuck some money at being able to pull "better" caliber or more women? The American Dream has reached the bedroom—with hard work, any man can do whom he wants to do.

The positive spin: these are men working to develop themselves to be their most attractive and confident, and they will gain pleasure from the sex that will accrue and the relationships formed with women they might not otherwise have met. Men aren't as confident as they once were, the dating scene can be brutal, so anything that makes guys feel like the good version of themselves is to be welcomed—and it means women will meet a greater selection of men, not just the naturally cocksure.

Another view: these are men suffering from a misplaced sense of over-entitlement: that no woman should be unattainable. This turns women into targets who are supposed to respond to triggers that men have somehow fathomed will dictate what they will find attractive. With a whiff of misogyny, men are being primed to see all women as potential conquests on whom to deploy their tactics. All a bit Harvey Weinstein High.

Depending on whom I spoke to in the room, I lurched between the two: bouncing between therapeutic approval and queasiness at the sleaze. I can't say the mental barometer was working at its best, though, seeing as

I was somewhat preoccupied by what was looming after lunch. The move from theory to practice. At the height of Fashion Week.

MIAMI ADVICE

For a British bloke, the idea of walking up to a woman on the street midafternoon and having to chat her up with the aim of getting her phone number is a living nightmare. Committing armed robbery or heading on vacation to a war zone would be less terrifying. What on earth to say as an opening line? How not to sound like a complete jerk? Alas, with no direct flights from Miami International to Kabul that day, I had to tag along with Julien and a handful of pupils as they headed toward the pedestrianized area by Miami Beach for the putting-it-into-practice module.

Lincoln Road on a sweltering Friday afternoon. Women are going about their business: catching up with friends over coffee, popping into shops, flitting to Fashion Week events, and generally displaying no inclination to want to be bothered by men who are paying good money to learn how to bother them.

As a few of us skeptically hang back, Julien seeks to demonstrate that he's not all talk. He brazenly heads over to Starbucks where a woman is standing outside, walks up to her, asks her where she's from and gets chatting. Just as that's going well, another woman walks past on her way into a store—so he stops her and then brings her into the conversation. The classic technique of masterfully opening up the "set," engendering a spot of competition, and projecting that you're a guy who's at the heart of his own party. Lo and behold, within minutes the second woman then asks *him* for his number and what he's doing that night. Astonishing stuff. And achieved sober.

The acolytes are more of a work in progress, perhaps taking the behavioral tactics a little too literally. One virtually manhandles a bemused girl into an ice-cream shop in an attempt to show her who's the physical boss. Another, a small man, yaps like a Jack Russell on heat at a model all the way down the block but fails to get more than a weary, repeated shake of the head. Oh, how I smirked. Until I was sent off to do my own stranger bothering, and told not to return without a phone number. Similar to the moment just before you pull off a bandage, if you happen to be standing on the precipice of a bungee-jump as well.

The first girl I shuffle up to doesn't speak a word of English. She sounds Russian. I deploy my full repertoire—*glasnost, perestroika, pogrom*—but she remains impassive. I'm then directed, by Julien's elbow, to a pair of women who are sitting having coffee. One has a stroller. Neither has any time for me. Before I'd even opened my mouth, they raise a hand—traffic-cop style—to signal *Don't even think of approaching*.

Down but not out, I'm pushed toward two models, who at least don't raise any limbs at me. What then follows is two minutes of dire conversation, where all I can think to ask is where to buy socks around here, boring myself into submission, after which I turn to Julien like an injured player signaling the manager that he wants to come off the field.

With confidence shot to pieces, I make my final approach, to a waitress taking a break. After some initial confusion about where she came from—*Barcelona* and *Macedonia* can be easily confused—we manage a nice chat for a few minutes about the collateral impact of the civil war in former Yugoslavia, before I pluck up the courage to ask for a phone number. Which she actually gives me. I head off with a renewed sense of swagger and faith in the American can-do spirit. It was only when we ran into her again later that I noticed a wedding ring on her finger. She'd given me her number out of politeness. You wouldn't get that in Britain.

(By the way, checking for a wedding ring in an obvious manner can be an elementary mistake. The most surreptitious way of looking: if a woman is sitting opposite you, gaze at something to your left that's on the same latitude as her hand, then slowly do a panoramic sweep to the right to something that just seems to have caught your attention, thus ensuring you'll clock the hand without ever being caught flicking your eyes down at the ring finger.)

I left Miami with mixed feelings. In the weeks afterward, I did occasionally catch myself in bars or at parties still holding back from going over to someone I liked the look of. I could hear Julien in my ear telling me just to go over—*whose permission was I waiting for?* He's right. One of my best relationships came from plucking up the courage to speak to a gorgeous girl who'd walked into the pub, but only once fueled by two pints rapidly downed. How many potential relationships have men missed out on by not having the nerve to approach a woman? It can be achingly awkward, if not impossible in the wrong mood, to approach a woman cold. Particularly in Britain, where girls are wont to look as though you've kicked them in the shin when you go up to talk to them. In the US, some women are kind enough to dish out phone numbers just to avoid hurting your feelings. Any little tricks or confidence boosters to get men over that hump have to be a good thing.

And yet, there was something that didn't quite sit right about the guys who were just too "hungry." Using (and overusing) the techniques, not to meet the right person but as a way of improving their batting averages. And in doing so, turning women into opponents to outplay. What was this "hunger"? If I were to take a stab at pseudoanalyzing a roomful of guys I'd barely met who have no interest in my analysis, I'd say the hunger masked some latent anger. Not some direct anger at women—bar the routine scars and wariness that come from rejection and loss borne by most guys in their twenties or thirties. But a wider frustration and anger at not having, by this stage in their lives, the money, status, security, and futures they thought they would have had and felt they were entitled to. Thinking that they'd be a step up from the rung their fathers reached.

And one way to compensate—another outlet for that irrepressible masculinity—is sexual conquest. A short-term fix to prove your masculinity. I know I've been guilty of that. (Why "guilty" though? Why do we so easily slip into moral judgment around sex?) When work setbacks have left me sitting on the couch feeling sorry for myself—and not much of a man—how tempting it's been to ping out a flirtatious text, seeking that instant ego hit of an incoming WhatsApp ting.

Sex to boost self-esteem and assert our manliness is hardly a new male phenomenon. But apparently the link between sex and how we see ourselves became much more pronounced from the end of the eighteenth century, once the Industrial Revolution began driving a steam-powered train through our traditional pillars of masculinity.[2] Until then, some young men could rely on the patriarchal plot of land coming his way: his identity, role, and future income were all nicely assured. All this was swiped away by industrialization, creating a legion of disaffected men who found a new means to prove themselves: the women they were coming into contact with as cities took shape. So from the 1780s (a precocious forerunner to the unruly 1980s), across Western Europe and North America, there was a pronounced rise in prostitution and illegitimate births and a drop in the age at which men were losing their virginity (from twenty-five or twenty-six down to eighteen to twenty years old among working-class men).[3] I daresay had there been pickup courses teaching men how to pull more mill girls, they'd have done a roaring business.

There was something almost too industrial about the hungry guys taking down notes as though Coach could get them higher up the league. Call me a Luddite, but I still think there's a hapless artisan charm to not having a set game play for how you approach women. A while later, I found out that a lovely wedding I'd been to had actually been the result of a pickup course. The groom had been feeling a little short on confidence and gone to a course. Then two weeks later he saw a girl he liked at a party. Instead of holding back as he usually would have, he marched over (in the crab-like arc), got talking, hit it off, and lo and behold ended up getting hitched. Thinking that the wedding that wouldn't have happened—and any kids they might one day produce—without a spot of pickup artistry, I duly gave the pulling gurus the benefit of the doubt. And thought no more about it . . .

SOME MEMBERS OF A GROUP YOU DON'T WANT TO BELONG TO:

- The grand mufti Sheikh Sadik Al-Ghariani: Libya's highest spiritual leader, who helped direct the Islamist-led takeover of Tripoli[4]
- Omar Bakri Muhammad: the Lebanon-based cleric whose old group al-Muhajiroun praised the 9/11 hijackers[5]
- Geert Wilders: Dutch MP who called the Koran a "fascist book"[6]
- Dieudonné M'bala M'bala: racist French comedian convicted of condoning terrorism[7]

. . . until a few months later, when Julien Blanc was admitted to this august club. Along with the hate preachers and convicts (and many others), he joined the ranks of those who have been denied entry into the UK in recent years. The home secretary exercised her right to exclude those "whose presence in the UK is not conducive to the public good." Ahead of his proposed tour of Britain, video had surfaced of him seemingly shoving girls' heads toward his crotch as well as video (that he'd shared) showing his hands around women's throats.[8] Without any mitigating context being presented—which would be a tall order—it's certainly pretty unpalatable stuff.

#ChokingGirlsAroundTheWorld began to trend, a petition to ban him from the country that exceeded 130,000 signatures, and with a Twitter squall in full progress it was an easy political win for Theresa May to deny him entry. As a journalist who'd been to his course just a few months earlier, I was asked on to the *Today* program in the morning and BBC *News at Ten* that evening for an inside take on a man of whom *Time* magazine was asking: "Is This the Most Hated Man in the World?" (The Boko Haram general who'd overseen the slaughter of forty-five villagers in northeastern Nigeria that week didn't make the shortlist.) I said, in essence, that while he might not be a feminist's cup of tea, I hadn't witnessed anything on the course that crossed the line, but maybe the home secretary had seen something that she deemed so serious she had to ban him from the country.

In reality, I doubt she had. When a Twitter hunt is in full cry, hard facts and corroborating evidence are mere luxuries. The idea that we don't automatically have the right not to be offended gets trampled underfoot. I even copped a heap of vitriol for merely describing what I had seen with my own eyes. To ban someone from entering a Western democracy is surely a big deal, not to be dispensed on a whim. Yet Julien Blanc, who I believe has never been convicted of anything, was charged and judged by social media, with punishment handed down by an opportunistic reactive government. I'm not his biggest fan, there are elements of the whole approach that make me queasy, and those photos looked a shocker. But surely the answer would have been to let him in, and if he infringed any law, *then* get heavy.

All this, just to go on a date.

FOOTNOTE: Julien Blanc went on to reinvent himself as a self-help speaker and transformational coach. Theresa May went on to become prime minister of the UK. He appears to have not yet claimed credit for her transformation.

4

YO! SUSHI DATING

CHEWING OVER ATTRACTION,
SEX, GUILT, AND COMMITMENT

No gentleman should permit a lady, whom he likes, but does not love, to
mistake for one hour the nature and object of his intentions. Women
may have some excuse for coquetry; but a man has none . . . Such blun-
ders, which may lead to one of two results. Either, having engaged the
affections, and excited the hopes of the lady, you will feel compelled to
marry her, or you will be disgraced, possibly cow hided, or shot.

The Illustrated Manners Book, 1855[1]

I daresay the prospect of being whipped by a leather braid, or even shot,
would do wonders to focus a guy on whether he might be leading a woman
on. Maybe Julien Blanc could have just been cowhided by Theresa May at
Heathrow arrivals. Such mid-Victorian chivalry, with its zero tolerance,
may be perfectly laudable. But were a single gentleman from the 1850s to
land in the midst of today's dating scene, he'd be arriving on an

unrecognizable planet. Metaphorically, he'd find himself in the midst of a conveyor belt–driven, Japanese-inspired restaurant franchise.

Dating for a man these days is like being stuck in YO! Sushi. It is to be sitting before a never-ending conveyor belt of options, constantly replenished by the swipe of a Tinder finger. New tasty-looking dishes appear, old ones come around again and momentarily look appetizing, friendly benefit plates stop you from growing too hungry but never really hit the spot. The choice is overwhelming, and it's too much fun to leave the seat even when you're feeling full. You stack the plates out of eyesight to deny to yourself how many you've had. You open your mind to trying dishes you've always turned your nose up at, but you know all along they are never going to work out. Then at some point you look up and realize that everyone else has left the table to settle down, move to the suburbs, and procreate. You think long and hard about the ones that have passed you by. You wonder whether the tastiest plates have all been and gone. And all along, you've been just another dish yourself—going around the conveyor belt for women to inspect. Oh, for some good old-fashioned sexually repressed Victorian etiquette!

Choice and expectation are terrible dining companions. And ones that, fortunately for the survival of the human race, man hasn't been dogged by for most of his time wandering around earth. Our foraging ancestors would go for months without seeing people outside their own tight band. In their entire lives, they might meet a few hundred fellow humans.[2] So they'd have to find a mate from the 150 or so women they'd encounter in their whole lives. I can swipe through that many in five minutes on my iPhone. Too much choice is crippling. If having more varieties of jam on sale in a supermarket can leave us floundering—and lead to a tenfold drop in sales once more than three jars are on offer—how can our brains cope with a bounty of what is supposed to be the most important selection in our lives?[3] If the choice was bad enough from just living in superpopulated cities, it is now dizzyingly augmented by the millions of available women and men online. How can you shout "Stop the clock!" when, if only you'd hung on a bit longer, someone better suited might have come around the corner or popped up online? And men don't have that same ticking biological imperative to kick your ass into pragmatic decisiveness.

Choice itself can be far more debilitating than accepting a fait accompli; deciding whether to move jobs or end a relationship is the stuff of nocturnal churning. This isn't a paean to arranged marriages; the enviable divorce rate of 3 percent or so in India is, I'm sure, testament to the stigma attached to separation and a dearth of gender equality. But I do wonder if, forced to make a go of it with some exes, you'd have just found a way of making it work out.

Too much choice creates fertile ground for the other unwanted dining guest to take root: the delusion of perfection. The longer you've held out, the harder it is to walk away from the buffet for good. To change table metaphors, having waited so long, you're holding out for a royal flush before going all-in (odds of 649,739 to 1 per hand).[4]

I know my dating expectations have been wildly unrealistic over the years. I berate myself for every time I'd walk away from a date thinking, *She was lovely, but* . . . I know the odds of a full house—sexiness, intelligence, humor, kindness, same city—are somewhat slender (a mere 693 to 1). What that great viral video plotting the Hot–Crazy matrix of women would classify as firmly in the nonexistent Unicorn Zone:

Below a five *crazy* and above an eight *hot* is your Unicorn Zone—these things don't exist. If you find a unicorn, please capture it safely and keep it alive because we'd like to study it and see how to replicate this.

My great-grand-foragers wouldn't have lost too much sleep over whether their partners were above-eight hots; ideally, they might have ended up with someone they vaguely liked the look of. But *they* wouldn't have been blanket-bombed with airbrushed images of unattainable women all their lives. Their notions of beauty would have been realistically rooted in the scores of women they might have met on their limited travels across a lifetime. Today, a man can easily be exposed to six hundred ads a day[5]—of which you can safely bet a decent proportion will feature models who have been shot in artificial light and touched up in Photoshop (having already been drawn from the pool of the exceptionally beautiful to start with). All of this scrambles the male brain trying to get a grip on authentic attraction (and let's not forget the impact this is having on women, who have these fictitious creations thrust in their faces as ideals to strive for). Everyone's confidence takes a kicking. Men are left to question whether their partners might not be objectively attractive (enough); women who go within ten feet of a magazine are made to feel miserable. It's a shitty deal for all of us. Let's banish this faux beauty and all smear ourselves in Dove soap—which undertook a campaign using real women, not models.

Modern dating expectations run amok not only in terms of our prospective partner's physical appearance but also in the very essence of what a relationship should be. If somehow you'd managed to avoid growing up with any film, TV, or mass culture, what would you expect from a relationship? Based just on what you'd seen of your parents and other families, you might hope for someone to share the chores with, some companionship and support punctuated by moments of laughter, anger, and an awful lot of everydayness. What you wouldn't expect is an ever-present giddiness from how happy your relationship is making you—a euphoria that can only be conveyed by a Hollywood score set to soft-focus visuals. No wonder it's so tempting to stop dating someone on the grounds that you're just not *feeling it*. Or, heaven forbid, because there are prolonged periods when it's all terribly mundane. *Where's the orchestra gone? Why aren't I feeling something more?*

There might be some wisdom to be drawn from the arranged marriage here (note: "arranged," not "forced" marriage—with families teeing up matches). Under our (fairly recent) model of marriage based on romantic love, we expect bells and whistles from the outset. The psychologist Robert Epstein, who has been researching love in arranged marriages, says we should instead maybe look to India, where the motto is: "First comes marriage, then comes love."[6] Love is something to be built over time—and, in the end, can actually exceed the happiness of those who married for romantic love.

Indeed, Brian J. Willoughby, from the School of Family Life at Brigham Young University (a Mormon institution not so hot on premarital sex), says this arranged approach can work because it "removes so much of the worry and anxiety around whether 'this is the right person.'" He notes, "Arranged marriages start cold and heat up and boil over time as the couple grow and get to know each other. Nonarranged marriages are expected to start out boiling hot but many come to find that this heat dissipates and we're eventually left with a relationship that's cold."[7]

Or sitting at the sushi conveyor belt prodding cold chicken teriyaki, or wondering whether to reheat the miso soup. When in fact I should slowly be savoring one dish that could, in time, be the basis for a delicious meal. A dish that has been carefully suggested by my parents who know that it comes from a nice dish family with compatible values.

It's easy to entirely embrace the innate wisdom of this approach, one that's still the basis for the majority of the world's marriages. Yet it's almost impossible not to feel the balls shrink just a little when a relative says, "I've found someone nice for you."

Dating itself is a relatively new phenomenon. The idea of going out with someone without any parental interference took off shortly before 1920 in the United States.[8] Until then, young men and women in places like Massachusetts had to make do with supervised house parties at which dancing was forbidden (too sinful) but kissing games were somehow waved through.⁹ What was once a structured activity, with its implicit codes and mores to push against, is now a baffling free-for-all that sits right on the fault line of shifting gender relations. Fifty years after the second-wave feminism that began in the sixties, it's harder than ever to delineate distinctly "male" and "female" dating behavior. Which is no doubt a good sign of progress; men have been too eager to dictate to women what their sexual desires are and should be. Yet some of the vestiges of "courting" awkwardly endure alongside this egalitarianism.

When, during the occasional blue moon, and generally only when in straight-man-starved New York, a woman hands you her phone number, it's slightly bewildering and deflates some sense of the chase. When the bill comes on a dinner date, you don't want to be seen as a controlling 1970s man by diving in to grab it, even when you have every intention of paying; moving the hand to wallet at just the right pace to convey *I'd like to treat you to dinner but don't worry, I don't want to disenfranchise your hard-won right to vote.* And it is a slight shock to the male system to be "used" (poor lamb) by a woman for sex. I once rolled over for a post-coital hug with someone new I quite fancied only to find she was having none of it. Orgasm (allegedly) achieved, she was up and off, leaving me to feel like the clingy one and get a taste of my own male medicine. These are just the slightly baffling wrinkles left over from generations of male dominance, and I'm pretty sure we won't implode as a gender as a result of these harridans making the first move. (I'm OK with it now, by the way, if you're a terribly hot woman who was about to poke away on Facebook.)

If *absurdity* could be fatal, though, then I'd fear for the future of mankind, thanks to online dating. A minefield of madness, incomprehensible human behavior, and inane hours you'll never get back. The antithesis to bespoke dates lovingly procured by family members and given time to grow and nurture with the community's support.

Online/app dating is to be stuck in an endless episode of *Miss Marple*— and about as erotic.

Each swipe of Tinder throws up a new riddle to solve: will this person look anything like their photos? Does the forced smile mask views on immigration that would make Donald Trump blush? And, ultimately, are they worth giving up two hours of prime box-set time to actually meet up with? Dozens of snap investigations conducted in mere minutes. Taking a whole episode to solve who killed the colonel in the vicarage looks like the height of analogue apathy by comparison.

When a profile starts to emerge as a real rival for box-set affection, the examination becomes increasingly forensic. You quickly learn that a profile with a single photo is highly suspect. Ditto only black-and-white photos. Only headshots raises a red flag. The more advanced practitioner will look to the (apparently indicative) upper-arm size. Relative height compared to friends. A disproportionate ratio of beach shots (narcissist). No smiling photos (get over yourself). More than one baby or puppy co-opted to project cuteness (overcompensating sociopath).

But this is a crude science. For all the rudimentary forensics, things have not always gone quite to plan over the years of online/smartphone dating. I was once forced to reveal on a radio show . . .

MY MOST AWKWARD INTERNET DATING MOMENTS:

10. The starer. She sat and stared for a full thirty-five minutes without asking a single question or answering anything in a full sentence herself. And she'd dyed her hair red two years before—but hadn't bothered to update her profile photos.

9. The "off-duty" high-class escort, whose profession only came to light (fortunately early on) when I saw her "review" page on her open laptop.

8. Spicy breath. Breath to make the eyes literally water—kept the face at a perpetual forty-five degrees to hers to avoid a direct nostril hit. To avert the risk of fainting, I had to take emergency measures and went to the john to download an app that faked a work phone-call ten minutes later.

7. The stripper who revealed she'd left her four-year-old kid at home. But don't worry, the neighbors have a key.

6. The woman who turned up from miles away whose first words were "Oh, God, you don't fancy me." She was kind of right. But she did do me a painting depicting how miserable my life was in London. Also kind of right.

5. The girl who came from many more miles (and continents) away, only for us both to discover that Skype chemistry abjectly failed to translate in real life—but we stayed friends and she didn't give me any paintings.

4. The S&M enthusiast who asked me to be her master, grossly overestimating the energy of a man in his late thirties.

3. The closet racist who'd have come across as more racially liberal if she'd arrived to the pub with a pointy white robe and burning cross. I walked out midpint after she declared she didn't like the look of black people.

2. The six-minute passive-aggressive life-coach date. Her opening words were "This isn't a date," despite us meeting via a dating site. She then ordered hot water, reinsisted it wasn't a date, and told me I wasn't remotely funny. I lost the will to live and was out of the door in under six minutes—after paying for her hot water.

1. The stunning but deliciously bonkers model who came from Germany to stay—twice. After it went pear-shaped, she just happened to move from Germany to a few streets away from me . . . and just happened to claim that she'd converted to Judaism without previously mentioning it to me. The last time we had dinner she told me

the funniest thing had happened to her on the subway that day: she'd seen aliens in the subway car. On the Bakerloo line.

Such are the perils of CSI dating.

FUTILE ATTRACTION

It takes no more than eight seconds to know if I might like someone on a date. Not a friend of a friend whom I've seen around or woman I might have run into at work. Rather, a cold date—say, from Tinder—whom I've never met before. This ridiculous sub-100-meter judgment obviously speaks immense volumes about my superficiality—a charge I don't contest. But whopping caveats about sweeping generalizations aside, I'd argue that men tend to have a fairly limited bandwidth for how much a woman can grow on them from the base starting point. It's rare to find a man who might say that he didn't find a woman (or man) at all attractive when he first met them but now he's really smitten by them. Whereas I have a number of female friends who attest that they didn't initially fancy at all the guys they have ended up with. The female room for maneuver seems far more generous and open to transformation by getting to know someone's character. This, to some extent, does happen for men: you might fall for the colleague you've really gotten to know over time, but I'd posit that, when pushed, you wouldn't have said she was entirely unattractive in the beginning. There are women I've known over the years whose character I adore but whom I could never imagine wanting to lean in and kiss. I've even fantasized about how taking X's character and Y's looks could create a perfect match. Yes, not the most edifying thought to think.

Are the women—and those guys—who have greater capacity to allow attraction to grow as personality shines through *better* people? Well, before you begin self-flagellating over your shallowness, it is worth looking at recent research published in the *Journal of Personality and Social Psychology*. It found that when looking for a short-term partner, women are just as prone as men to putting a high value on physical attractiveness. We're all superficial when it comes to flings. Moreover, although men do indeed "tend to more highly value physical attractiveness in long-term, committed relationships," women "tend to place greater value on social status" when it's looking serious. So while we're sizing up their bodies, they're checking out our social statuses. Which all makes crude evolutionary sense.

In our defense: "Men may have evolved to prefer romantic partners who appear sexually mature but youthful and are thus more fertile (short-term) and able to bear more offspring over the lifetime (long-term). Indeed, physical features linked to youth and fertility, such as smooth skin, soft hair, and a low waist-to-hip ratio, are especially attractive to men."

Whereas, pity the poor guy without a pot to piss in. "Women may have evolved to value social status in their long-term mates, as social status is associated with access to resources."[10]

At least if he's good-looking, he might get a few one-night stands, though.

Whenever I've ended up on one of those dates where your heart sinks—when you know immediately you just don't like the person but there's a minimum of forty-five minutes' small talk before an acceptable exit can be negotiated—who knows what physiological cues I had subliminally picked up on? Not just the obvious traits like height, weight, and eye and skin color. Psychologists have found that spouses tend to resemble each other slightly yet significantly in a whole host of less noticeable traits, including length of earlobe, distance between eyes, wrist circumference, lung volume and, especially, middle-finger length.[11] That's a lot to process in those eight seconds. (Character traits tend to align, too, with couples often sharing the same religion, ethnic background, socioeconomic status, and political outlook.)

Of course, if we are drawn to those who resemble us, it does mean that attraction is a subjective matter (another reason for magazines to stop pushing a homogeneous idea of what beauty looks like). The scientist and author Jared Diamond recalls a conversation about women and sex he had when camping with some men of the Fore tribe in Papua New Guinea. He reports the typical views of one man of the tribe:

> White women are unspeakably hideous. Just compare your white women with our women to see why—white skin like a sick albino's, straight hair like strings, sometimes even hair colored yellow like dead grass or red like a poisonous snail, thin lips and narrow noses like axe blades, big eyes like a cow's, a repulsive smell when they sweat, and breasts and nipples of the wrong shape. When you get ready to buy a wife, find a Fore if you want someone beautiful.[12]

And I thought I was fussy.

Were I to spend an evening camping with the Fore, once we got past lamenting the lost tradition of eating one's dead relatives (cannibalism was only outlawed in the 1950s), I might regale them with my own subjective five telltale signs for whether you genuinely like someone:

1. Do you enjoy kissing them sober?
2. Do you like how their T-shirt smells after they've worn it? Trust your nose (pheromones indicate a complementary immune system to strengthen any future kids you might have).
3. Could you imagine going to buy cupcakes with them on a Saturday while holding hands?
4. Do you overanalyze their texts for response times and how many Xs are deployed?
5. Do they look good in a hat? Don't know why, but this nails it even more than the middle finger.

OPPORTUNITY KNOCKS

Man has never been shy in the face of sexual opportunity. Those raucous 1780s—with their rise in illegitimate births and fall in the age at which men were losing their virginity—may have been fueled by young men moping about the loss of the family farms that were going to be their steady income and source of identity. But the mopey men entering the industrial era had newfound sexual opportunities by which to vent their angst in the emerging cities, full of property-less (hence vulnerable) women, professional prostitutes, and, for the middle-class man, servant girls to be seduced at home.[13] By the early nineteenth century, those live-in servants were just too much to resist for the men of the house: a quarter were dismissed for becoming pregnant.[14] Toward the end of that century, the posh young men of Delaware coined a term for the lower-class girls they now had access to in their pursuit of sexual gratification: "the chippy." One recalled that they "raided the amusement parks or the evening streets in search of girls that could be frankly pursued for their physical charms"—what they called an "old woman hunt." As for the women being hunted: "Her pretty face, her shapely limbs were all there was to a 'chippy.'"[15]

The author then went off in 1896 to Yale. Where, funnily enough, the Delta Kappa Epsilon fraternity was banned for five years in 2011 after members shouted sexually charged chants including "No means yes!" on a residential quad.[16]

But back to men and sexual opportunism. Given today's megapopulations, the explosion in online dating, and female desires more emancipated from male-imposed constrictions (though *slag* vs. *stud* disparities still persist), does this mean single men are living through a dream time of sexual opportunity? For the shy guy: surely some relief at not having to make the perilous trip across the dance floor now that initial contact can be struck up online? For the "hungry" guy: is there now a bounty of options on which to gorge? Does the roughly five quarts (a gallon plus) of semen a minute released across Britain, which would equate to around six gallons a minute in the United States—thanks to the Cambridge University statistician David Spiegelhalter for working that out[17]— represent an upsurge in action? The figures gleaned from the General Social Survey show that the average number of sexual partners has not significantly changed since the late 1980s. Indeed, even college students are not having more sex—but choosing the likes of friends rather than partners to sleep with. But *some* women are having more sex than previous generations did. In 1990, around 3 percent of women had had more than fifteen partners; by 2016, this was up to 7 percent. By contrast, 5 percent of men have had fifty or more partners.[18] Some women are becoming more like men, and for horny men that's an offshoot of gender equality worth celebrating.

Where male opportunism really surfaces is when market forces contrive to make the single male a sought-after product. Men who survive major wars return to find a society skewed in their favor. Post–Second World War Germany saw a spike in out-of-wedlock births as twenty- to forty-year-old men took advantage of being outnumbered three to two.[19] As early as June 1945, the *New York Times Magazine* was fretting: "With half the war won, men are coming home to America, but not enough of them"—and cautioned that psychologists were worried that 750,000 women who would never marry risked becoming "neurotic and frustrated." A doctor writing in *Esquire* raised the possibility of bringing in a polygamous marriage system in the United States.[20]

The women of New York today might feel that polygamy has been introduced in all but name, such is the prevalence of dating multiple people at once, though it's something that both sexes have embraced. (Women reacting to men refusing to be exclusive? Liberated women just doing what they want?) But when I made a radio documentary in New York about the dating scene there—*Find Me a New York Jewish Princess*—it did feel that some of the post–VE Day hysteria still abounded. The *Huffington Post*, citing that there were 150,000 more single women than men in the city, declared: "Why NYC Women Should Consider Flying Across the Country to Find Men."[21] One website allows women to find out the breakdown of single men vs. women in each zip code in New York, with instructions on how to navigate the map:

> Step 1: Slide the slider to the left around a bit.
> Step 2: Get depressed, eat several cartons of ice cream while watching Netflix.[22]

This numerical deficit, inflating the stock price of men, is manna from man heaven. From what I saw and heard (from exasperated women who couldn't find a decent man willing to settle down), men are predictably taking full advantage of this. The overabundance of choice and self-regard means men in New York leave it later than almost anywhere else in the US to get hitched: half are thirty-plus when they first marry.[23] Playing the field well into your forties doesn't seem to raise an eyebrow. During my week's intensive dating there—strictly for work purposes—I anthropologically immersed myself into the native's multidating culture, teeing up three or so dates a day. On the surface, it appeared a familiar world: the locals seemed to almost speak English, gravity was still an operational force, a Starbucks on every corner. Yet, in reality, it was a different planet: women routinely returned smiles, females made the first approach, a number was even thrust into my palm. Dating, but not as we in the UK know it. Meeting up with smug British guys out there, the accent exchange rate seems to add 20 percent to their usual pulling weight (30 percent if Scottish). I'm struggling to think of any good reason why I've not moved there.

GUILT ON THE SIDE

Definitive statistics around something as private as sexual activity are about as reliable as the polls before a presidential election. (If you can't even admit to abandoning Hillary, what chance do you have of being honest about the amount of intercourse in the last four weeks?) Who knows how much sex men are really getting and how this compares historically? Would an ancient Greek chuckle pitifully at the eleven lifetime partners of today's baby boomer?[24] Was that sweet spot between the introduction of the Pill and before the advent of HIV/AIDS in reality a time of unfettered liberalism? And that 11.7 percent is just the mean. Some 6 percent of men aged thirty-five to forty-four in the Natsal survey reported more than fifty partners in their lifetime; two guys (and one woman) claimed to have exceeded 500.[25] It seems that for those who desire sex, there is ample opportunity.

Should this be something to celebrate? Why shouldn't a man on today's dating scene—having thrown off some of society's prurient shackles and taken up new options driven by technology—fill his boots? After all, we are the only species whose purpose of copulation can be entirely unrelated to reproduction.[26] Many a female primate tempts a male only when she is fertile—with an irresistible red, pink, or blue vaginal swelling.[27] Sex clearly has many purposes beyond procreation, though I wonder whether even on a safe-sex one-night stand the mind might have been subconsciously fooled into thinking its seed had been spread, hence helping to explain why men might not want to meet again having gotten their way (other than just being bastards).

Sex when you're not in a long-term relationship: upsides. It's an ego boost, an affirmation of masculinity. The animalistic pleasure of getting to explore the body and scent of someone new. The hardwired thrill of chase and conquest. Being in a suspended state of projecting your best, most attractive side, before they have the time and space to see your vulnerabilities and darknesses. Compensation for being single when others have someone who truly cares about how their day was. Potentially porny with someone you haven't just done the weekly shopping with. Having better dinner-party stories.

All this set against, and perhaps contributing to, increasingly relaxed attitudes toward casual sex. Acceptance of premarital sex has been steadily rising—from under 30 percent in the early 1970s up to 58 percent by 2012.[28] Despite this rise, there remains a not insignificant residual opposition to people who are having sex outside of marriage. Perhaps partly a hangover from the troubled, religiously fueled attitude to sex that persisted through much of our recent history in the West.

Certain groups of early Christians saw sex as inhibiting spiritual growth. Christian men in the second century AD reportedly implored surgeons to remove their testicles. The theologian Origen is said to have performed his own castration.[29] The idea that sex could be harmful to a man endured. In Elizabethan times, it was said that sex "harmeth a man more than if he should bleed forty times as much." By the seventeenth century, doctors cautioned that a single male orgasm was the equivalent to the loss of forty ounces of blood, a view that persisted into the nineteenth century.[30] God forbid the man who considered a little self-pleasure in Victorian times—"a filthiness forbidden by God," howled the Queen's own physician. Masturbation was said to cause blindness, acne, insanity, and even premature death.[31]

To save the nation's youth from this "self-pollution," help was at hand from a Michigan doctor, one John Harvey Kellogg. Having identified thirty-nine signs of masturbation (including bad posture and a fondness for spicy foods), Kellogg cooked up a plain breakfast cereal to help tame men's sexual ardor: and lo, Corn Flakes were born. If milled corn wasn't enough to keep a man from touching himself, Kellogg suggested anesthetic-free circumcision (for the pain to be a reminder of the punishment) and even suturing up the end of the penis with wire to prevent erections.[32] Lord knows how the good doctor would have felt when the Crunchy Nut variant of his cereal was launched. Though in a Victorian *Shark Tank*, I'd say Kellogg would have lost out to the morality campaigner who invented a device, to be worn by men, that caused a bell to ring every time they got an erection.[33] An actual bell end.

After nigh two millennia of this sexual opprobrium bubbling away in the background, is it any wonder that we might just be carrying some of that judgmental baggage around, even within ourselves? And, it's worth noting, this condemnation-cum-sadism was just for *straight* men. One can only imagine the historical oppression heaped on gay men—until the nineteenth century, they could be executed in America; World War II code-breaking hero Alan Turing was chemically castrated in Britain in 1952—who have yet to fully shake off the vilification, still fighting for the likes of same-sex marriage in parts of the West. Or indeed on women, on whom genital mutilation, inflicted to avert sexual behavior, is anything but a historical quirk for many.

Some of this enduring reticence about casual or semicasual sex might partly be a cultural hangover, then. But, whatever carnal and emotional pleasures are associated with singleton sex, it's far from being the lush green grass some long-married friends may see when peering over the fence. Downsides: no idea what someone's sexual history is; accidental knocking someone up; sperm-stealing (I once encountered a woman who tried to talk me out of using a condom despite her not being on the Pill—*I wouldn't mind a baby and you seem like a nice bloke*); risk of mortifying performance failure (greater risk when you really like someone; women, take it as a compliment if you should be on the *non*receiving end); the sheer time and effort that goes into meeting and mating (energy that could be harnessed to, say, win a Nobel prize with time to spare); finding the mind drifting midaction to wondering whether the chase was actually more enjoyable than a sometime perfunctory experience; being racially misprofiled (I was once bafflingly asked, "What's it's like to be with a *white* girl?"); the hollow feelings that can sometimes follow. Indeed, dating can be a Darwinian dog-eat-dog world that doesn't bring out the best in your character. In the view of some sociobiologists, the male desire for variety and the female urge for security have turned seduction into an adversarial "sexual chess game."[34] And in its own way, chess can be brutal.

Your heart can be in the right place, even if your penis isn't.

THE FISH COURSE

And, ultimately, can too much casual or dating sex make it harder to settle down? Maybe too many wild oats being sown can tip the scales from helping you to get something out of your system to making you become too attached to the physical and psychological hit. Too many visceral memories in the bank to settle into a life of one steady joint account.

Is there, then, an optimal time to step away from the table and hang up your pulling boots? Strangely, mathematics might hold the key. What once was known as the "secretary problem"—how to work out which assistant to hire out of all the applicants—has been co-opted for the world of dating as "optimal stopping theory." An equation to tell you when to cash out. The theory dictates one must allow for an initial period when you're playing the field and getting to know the marketplace, rejecting all those in this period, and then you must be poised to grab the next best catch. According to mathematics lecturer Dr. Hannah Fry, in essence:

- Decide how long your dating window will be. That is, if you start dating at fifteen and want to settle down by the time you're forty, your window will be twenty-five years.

- Reject anyone who comes along in the first 37 percent of that window, i.e., in this case, until you are twenty-four-and-a-quarter years old.
- Then pick the next person who comes along who is better than everybody you've seen before.

It's not without its risks—such as letting an early dream sweetheart pass by—but, she maintains, it is "the best possible way to maximize your odds of finding your perfect partner," and one that happens to be exactly deployed by certain types of fish.[35]

Math wasn't my forte. But it doesn't take a (part-plagiarized) B at high school to work out that my 37 percent is well and truly in the rearview mirror. Perhaps I can proffer my own "emergency stopping theory":

1. When more than half of your closest male friends have gotten engaged . . .
2. . . . Settle down with the next person who comes along with whom it wouldn't be a total disaster if you happened to get her pregnant.

Perhaps there should just be financial instruments to cajole men into commitment. Parking fines at the buffet for overstaying your welcome. In late seventeenth-century England, when there was a perceived male shortage of ten men to every thirteen women in London, men, of course, dragged their feet. Exasperated by men's delaying marrying them, a group of women petitioned Parliament in 1693, calling for an annual tax on all men who remained single after they turned twenty-one.[36]

I'd be skint. But maybe happier.

5
RELATIONSHIPS. OH MAN!

THE MICROSECOND OF MALE HONESTY

A man is at his most sane the nanosecond he comes.

Once the bulbourethral glands crank into action, logic, reason, and maturity have their chutes on, ready to jump. The instance that first microglob of seminal fluid hits the urethra, sanity-inducing chemicals start their lightning advance on the brain. Down the man highway, spermatozoa wave with war-torn relief at the liberating forces of sense flowing in the other direction.

As soon as the testes start to refill, a man's judgment begins to become impaired again. The utterances of a man walking around with an overfull tank should be accorded the same respect as the pub drunk breathily declaring he knows how to fix immigration policy.

This is not (just) the stuff of an overlingering schoolboy mind. The latest thinking in the world of behavioral decision-making suggests that sexual arousal has a serious impact on our judgment. Being turned on is "analogous to the effects of alcohol."[1] You have to salute the dedication of Professors Dan Ariely and George Loewenstein for the lengths they went to in order to come to this conclusion.

A group of male students at the University of California, Berkeley, were paid $10 each to answer a series of questions about their tastes and behaviors. So far, an easy few bucks. But some of them had to answer the questions on a computer while "self-stimulating" with the other hand to a "high but sub-orgasmic level of arousal." To maintain the experiment's credibility, "subjects were instructed to press the tab key if they ejaculated, which would have ended the session."

Fortunately, self-discipline reigned at Berkeley, and the professors were able to demonstrate that sexual arousal has a strong impact on judgment and decision-making. A mere 42 percent of the nonaroused professed to find women's shoes erotic, which jumped to 65 percent among the aroused. A willingness among the young men to imagine having sex with a sixty-year-old woman trebled (from 7 percent to 23 percent). And there were even marked rises—among those touching themselves to non-tab-button levels of excitement—in those considering having sex with another man or an extremely fat woman, and those being able to imagine getting sexually excited by contact with an animal (alas, there's no data for the hat trick).

Should you be pooh-poohing this, that may say more about the current location of your hands. "We anticipated that people who were not aroused would underestimate the influence of emotional arousal on their preferences and decisions," reported the professors. If, for some reason, you should be self-stimulating while reading this, feel free to nod along.

Walking around with full testes is to be stuck in a potentially judgment-affecting state of arousal. If having a few strokes can be enough to make you more likely to grab a granny or caress a cat, then could full balls tip you over the edge into believing that there definitely are WMD hidden away somewhere or that Ukraine sure as hell belongs to you?

How many conflicts and terrible policies could have been avoided if government and UN votes had taken place in that sweet spot of post-ejaculatory clarity? It might be unpalatable to have comfort breaks at the

General Assembly just before votes, but the world would be a less crazy place. Perhaps strategically timed sperm donation drives could be instigated around cabinet meetings in Westminster, Washington, and the tribal area of North Waziristan.

For most of us, harnessing that window of sanity tends not to have profound geopolitical consequences. It's a moment of purity when our thoughts are sharp, unaddled by hormonal interference. A horizontal window of twenty-twenty focus. As we lie there, every sinew shouts either: roll over and hug (full Richard Curtis), mandatory peck and roll away with optional spooning (default relationship weekday), roll as far as gravitationally possible to the edge of the bed (perfectly nice but I need some shut-eye), begin instant manhunt for socks and pants for the getaway (*Will I never learn?*), silently lie there sending her taxi-calling alpha waves (*No, never*), or close the laptop with a head-shaking shudder of letting yourself down. *Sine semen veritas.*

These days, that window of lucidity screams only one thing: bring on the Richard Curtis. Walk away from the buffet, enough of this nonsense, time to find *that* relationship and settle down. But is this, deep down, what we, what I, really want? Am I just trying to fall into line, as the entry ticket for the next stage of life seems to require being in a relationship? Isn't committing to sharing the rest of your life/bed/holidays/dinners/genes with the same one person utterly terrifying for a man?

MAN VS. MONOGAMY

Samuel Pepys wrote a good diary. Incisive, descriptive eyewitness accounts chronicling some of the most momentous events in British history, such as the Great Plague and Great Fire of London sweeping through the capital's streets. An unparalleled insight into life in the Restoration. And the randy tendencies of a future Tory MP. Despite being married and professing love for his young wife, Elisabeth, Pepys rarely kept his pecker in his pants. Among others, there was:

- Betty Martin, the wife of a linen draper in Westminster Hall: "She has a very white thigh and leg, but monstrous fat."
- Mrs. Burrows, widow of a naval officer: "I had her lips as much as I would."
- Doll Powell, whom he "tumbled" with together with Mrs. Burrows one afternoon.
- Betty Mitchell, wife of an innkeeper: who did "hazer whatever I did."
- Mrs. Knepp, an actress: whose breasts he played with in a coach.
- Mary Mercer, a seventeen-year-old companion of his wife: whom he fondled while she washed his ears and cut his hair.
- Deb Willet, a waiting gentlewoman to his wife, who walked in on them mid-embrace: "And endeed, I was with my main [hand] in her cunny."[2]

The wife later went ballistic, threatened to slit Deb's nose, and wielded a pair of red-hot tongs at him. Historians draw a huge amount of information about everyday seventeenth-century life from Pepys's diaries, so it's perhaps fair to say that his sexual shenanigans weren't entirely unrepresentative: it seems well-to-do married men were prone to a spot of wenching. Indeed, this is borne out by the casual acceptance of the illegitimate children of the upper and professional classes at the time.[3] We don't know whether many were quite as prodigious in their groping as Pepys, who during the eight and a half years of his diary seems to have had sex with ten women and sexual encounters with forty more—all while married.[4]

Pepys was born into an era when men could get away with murder or at least the legal beating of their wives, who had no right to their own money and slender chance of divorce. In France, it wasn't until 1810 that married men were forbidden from keeping a concubine at home against the wife's wishes.[5] Throughout the great sweep of history, we've made the rules and skewed them in our favor and allowed a "flexible" approach to extramarital relations. But what if this is more than just a naked self-serving abuse of male power? What if the behavior across the centuries reflects something more fundamental: that the model of monogamous marriage just might not be suitable for many men? Am I craving a one-size-fits-all blueprint that's bust? Indeed, is it just our luck, of the last 150,000 years of *Homo sapiens* wandering the planet, to be born into a sliver of time when single-partner lifetime mating happens to freakishly be the norm? And then to be born in the West, not even landing somewhere like Saudi Arabia, where polygamy is possible and some good old-fashioned seventeenth-century divorce rules prevail (a woman needs the consent of a male guardian to divorce, yet a man recently divorced his wife over her alleged fondness for a camel over him).

Judged by its statistical results, marriage today isn't faring too well. The American Psychological Association estimates 40 to 50 percent of marriages won't make it. In Britain, 42 percent of marriages are expected to end in divorce.[6] A high school student turning in a piece of work that scraped 58 percent would be awarded an F.[7] So why do so many of us insist on signing up for this course?

That marriage is the default set text is no doubt partly due to the historical and lingering influence of religion, Christianity in particular. Ancient Judaism tolerated, but rarely practiced, polygamy, which it outlawed in the West in the eleventh century.[8] The Greeks and Romans allowed de facto polygamy through concubines and a spot of slave sex.[9] But Rome fell and monogamy spread. If Constantine hadn't converted to Christianity, would orgies to let off steam still be all the rage? In Pepys's England, theologians had banned the woman from going on top, the man from behind, any oral or anal, and advised against sex on a full stomach.[10]

It's hard to shake off centuries of dogma pushing marriage as the only moral option in town. And, often, the only legitimate way of getting sex. A man with balls full to bursting—especially if he'd been consuming Dr. Kellogg's advice—will sign up for anything, even arranging table planning at a wedding.

Just as religious influence waned, so the push for marriage has been taken up by a whopping "commitment industry." Weddings turn over an estimated $300 billion a year globally.[11] In the United States alone, 750,000 jobs depend on weddings: providing the food, drink, flowers, clothes, venues, photography, cars, haircuts, and so on.[12] Throw in another $40 billion or so spent on engagement and wedding jewelry—indeed, the very idea of the diamond engagement ring as de rigueur was invented by an advertising agency employed by De Beers in the late 1930s. Diamonds and profits entwined forever.[13] Another $40 billion for honeymoons.[14] Some $50 billion, say, for Valentine's.[15] Around $4 billion in online dating. And a mere $111 million annually grossed by rom-coms.[16] Totted up, that's a $434.1-billion-dollar industry, all predicated on men dedicating their penises to one vagina for their entire lives. If commitment were a country, it would have the forty-second-highest GDP in the world (just behind Sweden).[17] And there's nothing like a giant industry to dictate our tastes. The breakfast-cereal business, a modest $33 billion by comparison, has somehow persuaded us that shoveling refined sugar into kids' mouths is just what they need to start the day.[18]

Beyond the pressures piled on by religion and Commitment Inc., maybe the marriage model has also evolved for the wider benefit of society, if not necessarily for the experience of individuals. In the remote areas of Papua New Guinea, untouched by modernity and Hallmark, the surviving hunter-gatherer bands can give us some sense of how man lived for the last six million years. And it hasn't followed the rom-com script of boy meets girl. Rather, it's high-status boy meets a few girls—and some boys don't end up with anyone. This "mildly polygynous" state is, however, a recipe for tension and aggression. In those New Guinean Highlands, Jared Diamond notes, only disputes over ownership of pigs rival disputes over sex in triggering war.[19] Wiping out your own tribe fighting over women (or pigs) isn't great Darwinian business. And when it comes to fighting other tribes, monogamous societies can grow bigger and so raise larger armies, since low-status males aren't leaving to find themselves a woman elsewhere. Indeed, rulers wised up to this in the West; socially imposed monogamy emerged as a reciprocal arrangement, in which elite males allowed lower-ranking males to marry in exchange for their military service and tax contributions.[20]

The church. Big business. And now the army. All marshaled behind monogamy. A conspiracy theorist's wet dream.

MONKEY NUTS

Maybe the full weight of the military-industrial-religious complex has to be deployed given the scale of the task at hand: taming men's balls. Monogamy might not just run against how we might have lived for virtually the entire history of our species; is it also counter to our biology? To how we are wired?

The biggest clue lies between our legs. Should you have some scales on hand, you might find that the testes weigh around 1.48 ounces. Should there be a gibbon next to you, doing the same weigh-in, take pride that his nuts will be a mere 0.28 or so ounces. But any cockiness will be short-lived if there's a chimp lumbering up to the scales, with his big swinging 3.5-ounce testes.[21] We have bigger balls than a gibbon and smaller ones than a chimp—so what? Well, among our closest relatives, ball size indicates sexual behavior. Chimps need serious supplies of sperm to fuel their promiscuous lifestyle—and, literally, flush away their rivals' deposits. The male gibbon, on the other hand, is a monogamous sort of ape, spending his life with one gibbon wife and their offspring, eating figs and looking for insects.

He has no biological need for any larger testes, which would merely divert energy away from other internal tissues. Based on testes size, then, the human male would appear to be designed to veer toward monogamy but not quite get there—what some call being monogamish.[22] Indeed, the relative body size of human men and women anatomically indicates that we are geared to "mild polygyny" (one male and multiple females, just like another small-balled ape, the gorilla, whose testes weigh slightly less than man's).[23] No wonder, perhaps, that only forty-three of 238 societies across the world are monogamous.[24] And that extramarital sex has been reported from all human societies.[25]

The idea that man is fighting his biological software to fit into monogamous nuclear family units leads some sociobiologists to see this as the source of much modern misery and neurosis.[26] For all our trappings of civilization, we are basically great apes in cheap suits, sharing 98.4 percent of our DNA with common and pygmy chimps: all but 1.6 percent of our genes is just normal chimp DNA.[27] Indeed, chimps, like humans, are one of the very few animals to use sex for anything apart from reproduction: chimps deploy sex for multiple purposes, including building alliances and defusing tensions.[28] The chimp narrator in Will Self's *Great Apes* looks with pitying bewilderment at how humans have organized:

Humans often consort—and therefore mate—for life! . . . And while humans may display as much regard for their offspring as chimpanzees do, their perverse adhesion to the organizing principle of monogamy (perverse because it confers no genetic advantage) means that the gulf between "group" and community ties is a large one. Old humans are disregarded and neglected far more than old chimpanzees.[29]

It would take one ballsy husband to play the monkey card when caught cheating. *Sorry, honey, I had sex with that woman because my sociobiological instincts took over. Have you seen the comparative size of my balls lately?* We might be wired in a certain way, but our instincts don't dictate our behavior. If not, we'd be unable to pass a supply of sugar without gorging on it. We can settle disputes without resorting to aggression. Our diets aren't beholden to our dentistry. Some even choose to put their own quality of life above having children, which should run counter to every selfish-gene impulse. Individual human behavior around relationships is, of course, the product of a myriad of factors: the particular genes you've inherited, how you've been brought up, major life experiences, strength of sex drive, personal moral standards, the dynamic with your partner, what's going on in your work, health, mind, and life at any given moment, etc., etc.

The sugar cravings are a useful pointer, though. Where biological tendencies meet short-term pleasure hits, we are highly susceptible to overindulging. Look no further than the dramatic rise in global obesity: nearly one in three people on the planet is now clinically overweight or obese.[30] By being aware that we have this addictive-like predisposition to sweet things, rooted in a perfectly sensible survival mechanism for our hunter-gatherer bodies, we can at least factor that into how we run our lives. If we really wanted to keep obesity at bay, we would take the sugar out of kids' breakfast cereals, ban junk food ads on TV until after the 9 p.m. watershed, put fizzy drinks in plain packaging like cigarettes, and introduce a sugar tax, keeping this highly refined drug out of mind and reach.

Likewise, when it comes to sex, if you place a value on monogamy, then it's worth at least recognizing that there are genetic tendencies that might be pulling you in the other direction. I have friends who see these traits in themselves and take evasive action—like the sweet-toothed shopper who preemptively cuts out the candy aisle in the supermarket. I know men who, realizing they are prone to temptation, gave their wives their Facebook logins when they married, others who avoid situations where they might be drunk around single women, and one whose first reaction on receiving an out-of-the-blue flirty text from an ex was to show his wife the message the second it landed. These are men who know what they can be—or have been—like and don't dare risk the equilibrium that keeps the monogamy they cherish on track. These are what I'd call Category C guys in the sweeping classification of . . .

TYPES OF MEN IN RELATIONSHIPS:

A. The madly in love, who can't imagine even looking at another woman: prone to excessive PDA (public displays of affection, for the uninitiated among you), glazed-over eyes, and posting saccharine messages of love on Facebook. Genuinely excited to get married. Viewed with some suspicion/awe by other men.

B. The roving eye who would never act: a regular kind of guy who loves his partner but likes to think he's still got it. Likes a bit of safe flirting. Can be trusted in a strip club on a stag party.

C. The at-risk in the wrong circumstance: dedicated to his partner and doesn't want to stray but has traditionally been a bit of a dog. Can mitigate the risk of cheating by avoiding opportunity. Probably shouldn't get hammered in a strip club.

D. The plays away on "special" occasions: broadly monogamous and a committed partner but feels the need to let off steam every now and then, which he would see as no reflection on his feelings for his partner. Might stop short of full intercourse when letting off said steam. Sees the stag as the ritual giving him "permission" to let the inner chimp out.

E. The serial shagger: in a relationship but monogamy just doesn't work for him. Prone to affairs, flings, and maybe hiring prostitutes. An expert at compartmentalizing. Driven by the ape within that modern society is trying to constrain. His relationships may implode or sometimes function perfectly well in a nonconventional manner. Would be better off living in Papua New Guinea.

Type A is the gold-standard fairy tale, which I've only really felt in the first flushes when still high on oxytocin and often under the spell of an actress/singer who is still managing to pass off the fiction that she is a normal human being. B is probably the best grade that I—and most guys—can aspire to: romance that's rooted in reality. C would be a respectable pass. I prefer not to be in a relationship at all than be in one and stray. I don't want to be that guy who goes AWOL for a few hours on the stag, but nor do I rush to judge others who do. Who knows what's going on in someone else's relationship, what it takes to keep *it* together as well as a sense of themselves intact.

But judge we do when a man—or woman—is caught cheating. Political careers are ruined, celebrity love rats splashed across the front pages. A damnation that is driven not just by the extra sales generated by tittle-tattle, but a puritanical quasi-Victorian morality purveyed by the newspapers, which many of their readers, and scant few of their writers, would struggle to identify with in real life. In doing so, not only are papers trampling over people's private lives in lurid detail—making any chance of a couple putting the incident behind them that much harder—but they are also deterring anyone with a less than perfectly well-behaved libido from entering public life.

William Gladstone was a towering Liberal prime minister who took on the epic challenges of Irish home rule and Westminster corruption, yet he used to like to wander the streets of London at night, talking to prostitutes in an attempt to save them, before heading home for a spot of self-flagellation (and putting a little whip sign in his diary). David Lloyd George was an inspiring radical prime minister who tackled child labor and led Britain to victory in the First World War, though he also found time to earn the nickname of "the goat" for his prolific extramarital liaisons, including a mistress he kept for thirty years. Gladstone and Lloyd George wouldn't have lasted one news cycle—let alone four terms for Gladstone—under the scrutiny of today's tabloids—and we'd all be worse off for it. How close could Gary Hart have gotten to the White House in less prurient times? It's not to say that with great men come great libidos: there's evidence that accruing power in itself can lead to an overactive libido among men (and women) that can border on the reckless.[31] But if we want our leaders to have lived a little, to have flaws and empathy, to be human rather than vanilla party apparatchiks, then we might have to turn a blind eye to whom (rather than what) they are doing in office. If they have a decent health care plan or don't drag us into absurd conflicts, I don't care what politicians like to dress up as, or what they send photos of, as long as there is no power being abused in the relationship.

France used to have a fine tradition of Gallically shrugging off a politician's peccadilloes (the French mistress model = Category F). At President François Mitterrand's funeral, his wife stood side by side with his long-term mistress. Interestingly, a previous incumbent of the presidency, Félix Faure, is mischievously reported to have died while being fellated by his younger mistress. In more recent times, French magazines had the gall to publish photos of President François Hollande nipping out on a scooter in the night to see his mistress.

As that great Frenchman Inspector Clouseau said: "Anonymity is a virtue. Every fool knows that."[32]

What does it mean when a man has sex with another woman who is not his partner? Rather, what doesn't it mean? Well, it doesn't necessarily mean much—to him, at least. Sex can be entirely devoid of emotion. An ape-like animalistic act, though ideally lasting longer than the seven seconds taken by the common chimp to copulate.[33] The comedian Jerry

Sadowitz, in his act, talks about men needing a "sex wee"—an over-whelming physical urge, just like dying for a pee, though at least you don't have to negotiate with the toilet to sate that need.

This "need" of men was officially recognized by the British army in the First World War, which granted permission for soldiers to visit brothels (unlike the American troops, who, it was feared, could become exhausted by sex). Indeed, married men, who therefore were seen as being accustomed to intercourse, were given greater authorization for brothel visits. Officers, naturally, had their own separate whorehouses (red lamps for the men, blue for officers). And French troops were positively encouraged to visit a prostitute.[34]

No doubt the soldiers who returned home didn't love their wives any less, no matter what color lamp they'd cavorted under. I doubt there would have been much guilt, given the fact that in the century that had just passed, paying for sex was a rite of passage for the majority of men.[35] And this habit persisted: if the figure is to be believed, Kinsey reported that 69 percent of Americans in the 1940s had visited a prostitute. The Natsal survey in 2000 found that 9 percent of British men had paid for sex at some point.[36] The amount of paid-for sex has fallen but still persists. My only encounter with prostitution came when I was working as a young investigative reporter on the BBC *Six O'Clock News*, and I spent weeks trying to track down a sixteen-year-old Lithuanian girl who had been trafficked from her village to London. We eventually found her in a brothel near Heathrow Airport, the police raided it, and she was able to go back home to her distraught mom. It was grim stuff and indicative of the more exploitative end of the trade.

To get an insight into men who pay for sex with women—at the consensual end of the spectrum—I interviewed a middle-aged man, married for thirty years, on my old *Men's Hour* radio show. Mike had only ever slept with one woman—his wife—in his entire life, but then found himself working away from home a lot and began to visit brothels. That had then developed into a regular arrangement with one escort, whom he'd meet up with for dinner before having sex in a hotel. A mild-mannered, regular kind of guy, Mike was adamant that he loved his wife and his use of escorts was purely to sate physical urges.

"During sex we often experiment, doing different things that I don't do at home. For instance, I like to give pleasure to a woman, I like to give oral to a woman, and my wife doesn't like that. I can give oral sex to an escort, and that really turns me on. If I do it well and she has an orgasm, that makes me feel good, and I hope it makes her feel good." He also liked to dabble with the dominatrix side of sex and be tied up. Something that was never going to be on the menu with his wife of thirty years, whom I sensed tended to be a bit on the critical side.

"Kissing an escort is physically nicer than kissing my wife. They're professionals, they know how to kiss, and they don't complain about my kissing."

His wife eventually found out when he had an STD scare—he was using condoms for intercourse but not oral sex. Her reaction wasn't "overly pleasant," but, he says, "She understands that, when I was working away a lot, I did have some *needs*."

They are still married, and he is still seeing an escort, unbeknownst to his wife. That escort is Laura, a gregarious Irish woman and a passionate defender of sex workers. I interviewed her too. She said kissing Mike was "yummy," that she'd consider him a pal—though as to whether she felt he might have fallen in love with her, it was "no comment." As for the line of work: "Provided a client treats me with dignity and respect, we'll get along just fine. Sometimes it feels like work—when I'm tired and rundown—and other times I can't believe I'm actually getting paid for this. If a man is doing something I don't like, I tell him to stop. Just because he is paying, he doesn't have carte blanche; consent stands on its own.

"When I started off in Ireland, men would call from the country and say, 'I need to ask you to do something and I'm so, so sorry if it causes offense . . . but could we do it from behind?' This was exotic to them."

If a man like Mike wants to act on his urges, perhaps it is better for him to see a prostitute rather than find someone to have an affair with and maybe lead along and risk getting too attached or even caught. The arrangement has a transactional fence around it. Despite being busted, he still sees Laura behind his wife's back and says guilt never creeps into his mind. The closest he might get to it is: "Occasionally, I might sometimes think I'm spending the family's money on this."

Men can have emotionless, purely animalistic sex. But they can also not necessarily *mean* to cheat. (Yes, that does sound like another dire excuse, up there with *my balls are just too big*.)

As the Berkeley professors showed, an aroused man suffers from diminished rationality, akin to being drunk. In the cold light of day, he might well have no interest in having an affair; but once turned on, his rational sense is suddenly replaced by a strange fondness for shoes and grannies. Many a man has no *intention* of cheating. Indeed, one of the biggest factors in infidelity is opportunity: people falling into affairs rather than planning them.[37]

Opportunity used to come in the form of guys like Mike working away from home, but now it overwhelmingly abounds with social media. More grist to the mill for those Cat C friends who eschew Facebook and nightclubs—and, in one case, makes sure he regularly masturbates to keep the full-ball demons at bay. One guy in his midforties who had finally hung up some rather well-worn pulling boots to settle down, told me that while the concept of monogamy was "insane," what kept him faithfully focused was visualizing the prospect of another man one day having a say in how *his* kids were being brought up if he were to mess up. I have tried to adopt a similar Zen-like projection for fast food. I abhor McDonald's, but once every eighteen months or so I used to drunkenly crave that moment of the initial bite into the gherkin. But focusing on that burpy, greasy postburger moment (when the gherkin pleasure has morphed into the sensation of eating cardboard) just about releases enough clarity and willpower for me to walk past the stinky arches peddling their biological crack. With enough foresight, can you mitigate against that unmeant fling by meditating on how you'd feel the moment after release? Projecting to when you're lying there feeling wretched—or seeing some other guy telling your kids that their new football team is now the Cowboys?

GO APE?

So men can have emotionless, carnal sex. It can be an opportunistic slip, exacerbated by an addled mind running low on rationality. It can be booked a week in advance, with relish of the physical pleasures to come, and where any guilt, if it even exists at all, can neatly be compartmentalized away. (Or it can of course be the last thing that you'd ever do to the person you love most in the world.)

If an emotion-free, purely physical expression that allegedly doesn't diminish the love for our partner, taps into our biological software, is the norm in a majority of the world's societies, and is how man has lived through the vast swath of his time on earth—before modern Western religious/business/political interests imposed monogamy for their own benefit—then surely this raises the somewhat incendiary question: is it less serious for a man to have an affair?

Judging by penal codes throughout history—many of which are still brutally in place in parts of the world—the men (naturally) who set the rules certainly seemed to think so. Indeed, the Lord Chief Justice of England in 1707 described adultery by a woman as the "highest invasion of property" a man could experience.[38] Today, any argument over the relative severity of an affair would be somewhat less centered around the idea of invasion of property and more on the notion that female extramarital sex runs counter to their sociobiological instincts—that men are wired to seek variety while women want to look for security.[39] So somehow, that's a greater transgression. A more visceral betrayal when the woman is penetrated—when another man is allowed inside her and inside the sanctity of the relationship—compared to the idea of the man as a penetrator to something outside the union.

"Every time we have sex, I think about her with another man. I am trying my hardest to forgive her and forget about it, but I can't. What should I do?" one man begs of his church.[40] The idea that another man has been inside his woman is just too much for many to move past. "In general, men can forgive themselves for their indiscretions, but find it much harder to forgive their partners for the same," says the psychotherapist Phillip Hodson. "For a betrayed woman, an affair is an offense against her dignity. Whereas, for many a betrayed man, it's an offense against his manhood. The betrayal goes right to the core of his identity."[41] A hammer blow that can drive men to murderous rage. Some 1,099 wives or girlfriends were murdered in the US in 2010, compared to 241 husbands or boyfriends.[42] A Cardiff man killed his partner after she changed her Facebook status to "single."[43]

I know the pain of being cheated on. My longest relationship to date—in my late twenties, too early to appreciate what I had—finally imploded when I discovered that she had been having an affair with a colleague. Bizarrely, I'd had a premonition during a vivid bad dream on an overnight flight that she was seeing someone at work, and I confronted her when I got back to Britain. The pain when the truth came out: it's to be rendered winded, dazed, nauseous all at once—an all-consuming, hardwired rage. I stormed out and jumped on my rickety Vespa, racing down the Edgware Road at seventy miles per hour in kamikaze fury as the phone buzzed unanswered in my pocket. It's so visual, visceral, primordial. *Another man has penetrated my girlfriend.* It cuts deep into the tenderest, most vulnerable—most animalistic—part of what it is to be a man. Exhilaration and despair in equal measure.

Are men right to be less forgiving? To assume, perhaps, that somehow it is worse—that it has more meaning—when a woman has the fling? I gingerly raised the notion with a group of female friends over lunch. *A man can have utterly emotionless sex—it can mean nothing to him*, I posited. *So can we*, they all shot back. I persisted, running through people we knew and eventually agreed to settle that emotionless sex was 60/40 a male/female preserve among our cohort. I raised it with a guy who runs one of those affairs dating sites designed to enable married people to cheat. *Aren't men better at compartmentalizing their feelings?* It's the other way around, he said; it's the women who are pros at running separate mobile phones and never letting on.

If ever evidence were needed that women are able to put this away in an emotional compartment just as neatly, if not more so, than men, it's the prevalence of dads bringing up kids under the delusion that they are the biological father when they are nothing of the sort, while the wives keep mum. Naturally, there are few definitive statistics around this. One big study estimated that 4 percent of British men are "cuckolds."[44] Another extensive global survey reported 2 percent.[45] Historical rates in America and Britain have been put as high as 5 to 30 percent (perhaps partly due to a lack of contraception in the past).[46] Indeed, scientists in Nottingham in the mideighties noticed something was up when 23 percent of the women in their study whose husbands were sterile managed to become pregnant *before* receiving treatment.[47] (These women were having their biological cake and eating it, passing on their genes while having someone around to help raise the offspring.) The supercuckolded men of the southern Indian Nayar society, where women have multiple lovers, used to deal with this by raising their sisters' children, with whom they at least shared a quarter of the same genes. Some male fish don't take any paternity chances, pouncing on a female's eggs as soon as they are laid, then taking them away to fertilize and look after themselves.[48]

Elsewhere in the ocean, a male clownfish is swimming around minding his own business: keeping an eye out for a hostile stingray, maybe musing on the excellent symbiotic relationship it has with the tentacled anemone it hangs out with, puffed up with pride that Pixar chose to base *Finding Nemo* on his species. But our fish feels a stirring in his loins. The gonad wall starts to invaginate, ovarian tissue develops, and within a couple of weeks the testicular region has become small and nonfunctional. Nemo finds he's female. The underwater distinctions between male and female blur, with many a female fish ending its life as a chap. Onshore, to tenuously land this fishy analogy, we might say that there's a blurring of male and female sexual behavior: what can now be truly classified as distinctly "male" or "female"? To spend a week on Tinder is to surf a wave of sexual hermaphroditism. Men have lost their ownership of infidelity (if ever they really held it): in the United States, the percentage of wives having affairs rose almost 40 percent during the last two decades to 14.7 percent in 2010, while the number of men admitting to extramarital affairs remained the same at 21 percent.[49] In England, the amount of divorces granted due to adultery is now the same for men and women (15 percent).[50] While not great for the couples or any kids involved, on one level it could be seen as a positive, I guess: women throwing off the *Female Eunuch* straitjacket, economically autonomous and free to follow sex drives that are just as strong as men's.

But to return to the question I've been ducking: is it less serious for a man to have an affair? To step straight onto a gender mine, I'd argue that potentially there is a telling difference. Researchers have found that when men stray, it is more likely to be when they are feeling negative or fed up: it is a self-destructive, exhilarating act of defiance, up there with getting into a fight, drinking to excess, or committing a crime. Whereas, for a woman, cheating tends to be more a reflection of low relationship happiness and boredom.[51] In other words, for a man it's more a case of how he feels about *himself*; for a woman, it's how she feels about *him*. While an affair or a fling by either party could have profound consequences for the relationship, there is an argument that a woman cheating is more likely to indicate that something is seriously wrong with the partnership. Indeed, by the time a woman has had an affair, she may already have been mentally checking out of that relationship. (Whereas for the man who doesn't see an affair or a dumping coming, her cheating tends to be more of a bolt from the blue that leaves him a shattered, gibbering wreck.)

In my own case, after the rage subsided and I managed not to wrap my scooter around a lamppost, I eventually came to see my then-girlfriend's affair as just that: a symptom of how the relationship had derailed. It was dead in the water by then. While what she'd done was undeniably shitty, I took my ample share of the responsibility for really not putting enough into that relationship, brushing off the numerous "Where are we going?" talks, and being disengaged over the previous three years. But once spurned, I fought like a bastard to get her back. Flowers sent to work escalated into turning up at her flat, *Love Actually* style, with declarations of love written on big sheets of cardboard. When that failed, as a final throw of the dice, I snuck onto the same flight as hers without being spotted (the month before, I'd had to do the same to confront a murder suspect on camera—useful training) and sent a poem down the aisle to her via a flight attendant. At the very moment she received it, as I stood up to go in for the big romantic reveal, turbulence struck and I was sheepishly sent back to my seat before getting a word in edgewise. When we arrived at the destination—where we'd been planning to vacation together before it all went pear-shaped—she said it was the most romantic thing that had ever happened to her, but could I now please go back to London. Ouch.

In retrospect, I don't know whether it was the immediate fear of loss, mixed with an underlying sense of having created the conditions for it, that drove me to such lengths, and had we gotten back together whether I'd have been able to truly overcome her infidelity. Or whether I would always have felt that innate violation of another animal having invaded my domain. It's impossible to say. But the majority of people who discover a cheating partner remain married to them for years afterward.[52] Ironically, when, years later, she came to analyze her behavior, she ended up exploring what had prompted her to become so "male," as she saw it.

Talking about men's flings potentially being less "serious" is not to be flippant. An affair can be an incredibly destructive act that hurts the people you are supposed to love most, damaging yourself and causing children to see their homes broken up in the process. That young people today seemingly oppose cheating more than their generational predecessors perhaps reflects the first-hand pain of growing up in broken homes (good for teenage rebellion, costly for later therapy).[53] Rather, the point of taking an uncompromisingly frank look at men's natural instincts, how we've lived through time and across cultures, the forces that dictate what our norms should be (from the Church to tabloids), what sex can or can't mean to us, opportunistic slips, and our capacity to compartmentalize the physical from the relationship itself, is all because the model of monogamy is just so challenging for an awful lot of men and women.

In a world where a fifth of men in relationships are apparently having affairs and nearly half of marriages aren't going to survive, surely we need to lift the hood on what's going on for men. This isn't just about whether a man can keep it in his pants. This is about the entire challenge of the monogamous nuclear-family, lifelong-partner model. Sex is just a part of that picture. It might be a barometer for the wider state of a relationship but, depending on any given couple in any particular phase, it can be either a peripheral or a paramount issue. I've yet to find a sleep-deprived father with young kids who puts regularity of intercourse at the top of his things-to-worry-about list. Sex barely touches the sides of what we're up against. "It is a real experiment to try to bring together two fundamental human needs—our need for security, and our need for adventure—in one relationship, to ask the same person to make us feel safe and stable and make us feel playful, mischievous and adventurous," says the relationship counselor Esther Perel.[54]

Making this model, this experiment, work in today's society is a serious undertaking, navigating past some heavy-duty pressures. To deflect the projections of Hollywood romance that are pumped into our brains. To resist the temptation for instant resolution or dissolution during a sticky patch. To develop in tandem with someone when your cycles of personal change (maybe seven years) are out of synch. To spend more time together than marriage has ever entailed before; in Pepys's era the average union lasted only seventeen to twenty-two years (depending on class) before one partner died.[55] Note the huge rise in "gray divorce"—doubling among the over-sixty-fives in the States in a generation.[56] To maintain a sense of identity and who you were before being consumed by and regarded as part of a union (perhaps a big driver in those who stray). To physically be shut away in a domestic unit and detached from being a part of a wider tribe. To face down the expectations around modern parenting. To weather the storms unleashed by a dearth of work security—something that strikes at the heart of male well-being and affects how men function in relationships (which we'll look at later). It's significant that the share of working-class whites who say their marriages are very happy has plummeted to barely 50 percent—despite fewer getting married in the first place.[57]

These are nutty times to put on your best suit, stand in front of everyone you know, and publicly commit your penis to one vagina for life. And then celebrate with mushroom vol-au-vents.

THE WORST FORM OF COMMITMENT, EXCEPT FOR THE OTHERS

I have my own wedding registry list. Less a series of domestic appliances from Bloomingdale's. More a mental checklist that unwelcomingly barges into my brain every time I'm sitting in the pews watching a couple tie the knot: the fears that would have to be faced down for me to be able to stand where *they* are.

- How do you maintain sexual chemistry over a long period of time?
- Has there been too much previous chimplike behavior to take this level of commitment on?
- If the marriage were to split up, would the pain of separation not be off the scale?
- How can you face inflicting a divorce on your kids and driving them into a lifetime of therapy?
- What happens when you want to spend a night alone in your bed?
- Why do I have a friend who has to masturbate in the shower because his wife sees self-pleasuring as a betrayal?
- Who on earth could put up with me and the bullshit in my head for a lifetime?
- What happens if one of you changes and you actually stop liking each other?
- What happens if her parents insist on one of those awful hotel weddings in which the enjoyment factor is on a par with circumcision?

And people think I'm welling up at weddings due to the romance of the occasion.

Weddings themselves are the bane of the single person's life. The same table with the same other single pariahs, wedding after wedding. On high alert to make a Usainian bolt to the restroom the second the band strikes up for the first dance and invites couples to the floor: a sea of shuffling suburbanites. Having been best man 4.75 times (always the bridesmaid),

I've seen how—with the exception of those Category A doe-eyed guys—the day really has very little to do with the man. Mannequins in black tie who are wheeled around tables, pushed in front of cameras, and, like the old Action Man figure who spoke when you pulled a string in the back of his head, forced to parrot the same old line about how beautiful every female relative within a square mile looks.

Best man four times—and part-bestie at two other weddings. But "last man in" for about the same number of nuptials. I seem to have an unnerving capacity for girls to marry the next guy they date after me. Sometimes within months. It would only be fair, and certainly liven up proceedings during the stale chicken, for there to be a toast to the last man in. *Today wouldn't be taking place without the man who truly lowered my wife's expectations around relationships so that she's now willing to settle down with a shmuck like me. Raise your glass for the last man in!*

And yet. For all the fears that churn around, the statistical odds that something will go pear-shaped and doubts that this is even a natural state of affairs for a man, why is there a defiant yearning within me to settle down with someone? Why, when I very occasionally meet someone who has "full house" potential, does a giddy excitement build within? If the flop is starting to look good, I'm already visualizing what it would be like to parent together, having loving dinners at her folks' place where I'm welcomed as a son, going out with other couples to hot restaurants that have just opened: generally morphing from taciturn grunting guy into a moonstruck girl in *Glee*. OK, then the fourth card usually reveals overwhelming actress/singer narcissism and I painfully lose all my chips.

What's going on?

Brainwashing? Maybe. What's the free will of one man in the face of millennia of religious teaching and a multibillion-dollar Commitment industry? All reinforcingly seared onto the formative brain by seeing the adults in the society I grew up in pair off into couples. If I can be conditioned to see a bearded man with a blade lopping off a boy's foreskin at eight days old as perfectly acceptable—indeed, something to be celebrated with a smoked salmon bagel—then surely our norms are up for grabs. And we get a thrill in ticking off the perceived norms of success as we achieve them—degree, good job, house, wife, kids, comfortable retirement—just as we once might have got a kick from getting a good grade from a piece of homework. We're competitive creatures who like to pass or exceed at the Adulthood modules. So, yes, I would never dismiss the social osmosis that's directing my brain toward finding a life partner. God knows to what extent, just as God knows—if He/She exists—why I have no foreskin.

But in the here and now, what are the prosaic factors I can divine that make me and many a man want to embrace this superchallenging and arguably absurd model of lifelong commitment to one partner? In high school geography class, we looked at the push-and-pull factors behind migration: what drives someone to leave an area and what attracts them to go somewhere else in particular? I'd say that this is entirely analogous to settling down: leaving singledom and moving to a state of commitment. Where citizenship in this new state is marked not by a passport, but by an updated Facebook status and shared currency.

Reducing why you might want to spend the rest of your life with someone to a series of schoolboy push-and-pull factors isn't perhaps the height of romance, but it's good to at least know the rational underpinning for applying for a visa rather than just jumping on the boat.

PULL FACTORS—TOWARD SETTLING DOWN

Love: See, romance does get an appearance. The feeling of being in love can be the most amazing sensation. An endorphin-filled high of intimacy, a feeling that nothing in the world is insurmountable when you are together, an urge to buy presents that will really tickle them, a recognition that there is someone who truly carries your worries as theirs, where the sum is greater than the two parts. Who wouldn't want some of this?

At its best, it can become utterly central to life itself. The most inspiring example of love I've seen is between Kris and Marita Maharaj. Both in their midseventies, they've been married for forty years. He's spent the last twenty-nine of those locked up in a jail in Florida—including fifteen years on death row—for murders he is undoubtedly not guilty of committing. I've been investigating his case since being a cub reporter in local news and I've seen Marita give up everything to stand by her man. Living thousands of miles from their home and friends in Britain, subsisting on handouts from friends, just so that she can make the weekly trip to visit him in prison. At one point, those visits became noncontact—they were separated by prison glass. Her entire adulthood sacrificed to supporting her husband. "I married Kris for better or worse," Marita says. "I was with Kris when it was better, and I will be with him as long as it takes to get him out of this country." Her visits have kept him sane, and no doubt alive, during nearly three decades of trying to prove his innocence.

"My wife has been my backbone," Kris says, dressed in his pale blue correctional facility fatigues. "Without her, I wouldn't have survived. Seeing her are the happiest moments of my life since I've been here—they keep me going for the next visit."

Kids: I'm up for a spot of reproduction (something potentially more profound about fatherhood later on). And there's certainly a human biological imperative here to being part of a union. Unlike other animals, the human child isn't born able to fend for itself—so the odds of your offspring (and genes) faring better are improved by having two parents around. Inner Gibbon 1, Chimp 0.

It's good for you: A man in a good marriage is likely to live longer, enjoying up to 46 percent lower death rates from heart disease and surviving prostate cancer for nearly twice as long as a single man.[58] But you're better off staying single than going through a divorce. Those in the "warmest relationships" are also likely to earn more money: an average of $141,000 at their peak more than those at the chilliest end of the relationship scale. And they are three times as likely to end up in *Who's Who* due to work success.[59]

Sense of security: As the old securities that came with being a man—that job for life, guaranteed status, and purpose—have fallen away, it can be a choppy, harsh world out there. Being part of a team, fighting the daily nonsense of life together, rather than toughing it out on your own, is appealing. A trait we can see at play in the nineteenth century when work insecurity led to a new yearning for the care of a loving woman.[60]

Indeed, that may explain why the needle seems to be shifting slightly back toward marriage. A college-educated American man who married in the yuppie 1980s had a 20 percent likelihood of being divorced by the tenth year; that dropped to 16 percent for men married in the 1990s.[61] Those alpha-male 1980s saw a peak in the rate of men having affairs,[62] while during the recent economic recession male opposition to marital infidelity significantly rose.[63] When we're feeling economically insecure, a monogamous hug will do nicely.

PUSH FACTORS—AWAY FROM SINGLE LAND

Entry ticket: One day you find your access card doesn't work anymore. Without any warning, the codes have changed. Access has been denied to the next phase of life—unless you're part of a couple. Conversations become unrecognizable, peppered with phrases like *school zone*; social life retreats from the public to a private sphere of couples dining in rotation; some friends completely fall off the radar; and finding enough people to go on vacation with becomes a logistical challenge. You feel as if everyone else is orbiting on a different trajectory: they have graduated to the next level, which can only be accessed by embracing the partnership model. If I can feel this as a man with time hopefully on his side, I can only imagine how acutely alienating it might be for single women. Nor is it just a straight issue. A gay guy I sometimes work with told me how, as he gets older, he struggles to place where he fits into society, whereas couples with children can jump aboard a journey that drives them for the next twenty or so years.

Loneliness: The feeling of being lonely is something that would have been entirely alien to our hunter-gatherer ancestors.[64] Lucky buggers. To come through the door in the evening and know you're not going to talk to another human—unless you make a real effort—can be deeply dispiriting. It can sap the mood and make way for a lethargy that renders you beached on the couch, taking a Netflix hit. The wealthier we've become as societies, the more socially poor our lives are. For a man, there's a particular rub to the couples-centric lifestyle: you lose your pack. The band you've grown up hunting with will one by one desert you to live with their new nuclear clans, far away in some territory dictated by the Best High Schools ranking.

Again, this isn't just confined to straight men. Recently in London's Soho, a gay group convened to discuss "Overcoming Loneliness." It was brought together by drama therapist and director of *A Change of Scene*—a gay and bisexual men's discussion group—Simon Marks, who confessed: "I spent years on the scene struggling to live up to the gay ideal that we're supposed to live these amazing lives of sex and parties and fabulousness. That's just not been my experience." After a fruitless night cruising in a bar, "I walked through Soho and saw people drunk or with their boyfriends or having fun. Then it hit me. *I was feeling lonely.*"[65]

It's tiring: At some point, it just becomes way too tedious and tiring to go through the motions of singledom. Having to tidy the flat before a date in case it goes swimmingly, keeping ear hair under routine surveillance, taking unknown internet dates to pubs off the beaten track to avoid bumping into anyone you know, avoiding self-pleasure 24+ hours before a date to ensure a base level of motivation to get off the couch, and forcing yourself to approach someone you like the look of in case they happen to be *the one*. Conversely—perversely—there's a strange relief when someone seemingly attractive from a distance turns out to be less so when you get up close. Enough already . . .

No wonder a seventy-five-year Harvard study, which followed 268 men in order to see what makes people flourish, recently reported: "The seventy-five years and $20 million expended on the study points . . . to a straightforward five-word conclusion: 'Happiness is love. Full stop.'"[66]

ALL YOU NEED IS LOVE (MORE REALISM, LESS MORALISM, AND MAYBE A PILL)

Love, security, kids, less risk of keeling over with a heart attack, an opportunity to throw off the shackles of loneliness. But to taste these sweet fruits, there's only one real game in town: some sort of lifelong partner arrangement. There are no other mainstream models on offer. Sure, there's still the commune option—in one of the 2,571 "intentional communities" dotted around the world—but I can't help feeling that it would all end up with an accusatory note on the fridge for stealing someone's hemp milk. To paraphrase our greatest leader in the UK, maybe marriage is the worst form of commitment, except for all the others. And Winston seems to have been a devoted husband throughout his fifty-seven years with Clemmie.

If lifelong partnership is the game in town, can it be played differently? With one in three kids in the United States growing up without a father—and a million in the UK—is there any creative thinking to tweak the model? Something, for example, that would help alleviate any pressures of feeling trapped or losing your identity while still having a strong love for your partner?

Sex is an obvious place to start. That 65 percent of kids in the Riverside ward of Liverpool are growing up in homes without dads isn't simply the product of too much randiness; it's a reflection of a web of social factors, from generational deprivation to the impact of unemployment on male self-esteem.[67] But let's not entirely negate the inner ape: monogamy, as we've seen, can be challenging. So would a more honest and relaxed attitude to fidelity help? If we were less conditioned—partly through the eyes of tabloid sales–led morality—to see infidelity as so treacherous, maybe when it invariably happens to some couples it wouldn't feel like such a make-or-break moment. Would I have flown off into less of a high-speed rage if I'd been conditioned differently? A more honest, less moralistic media is needed then. Some of that Gallic shruggery. The exploration, as Esther Perel asks, of whether there is a nuanced distinction between "cheating and nonmonogamy."[68]

On an individual level, should "arrangements" be something that couples can more openly discuss? I know of several gay couples who have struck deals, effectively giving permission to cheat as long as:

- It's a one-night affair only.
- It's with someone they both don't know.
- It doesn't take place in their house.
- It's safe sex.
- The other partner never gets to know about it.

This model recognizes that there are *needs* but compartmentalizes the fling so that it is physically, socially, and emotionally detached from the relationship. A gay friend said that although he had such an arrangement in place during a three-year relationship, he never actually strayed: it was *knowing* that he had the freedom to do so, in theory, that was the thing he most craved. No doubt arrangements and open relationships are aplenty in the straight world too, with some people suggesting the numbers are increasing (though whether there are actually 15 million swingers in the US in more than just tabloid imagination is open to debate).[69] We live in unconventional times. Fewer than half the kids in the United States are growing up in "traditional homes," i.e., with two married heterosexual parents in their first marriage.[70] Perhaps we need to be open to, and be able to talk frankly about, less conventional approaches to accommodating the sexual urges, the *needs*, that a man and woman might have. Whatever it takes to straddle that tightrope between adventure and security—to be committed yet still able to feel alive—whether that can be achieved between the two of them, or with one or both of them having to look outside the relationship.

Unless we could all just get it out of our systems on one set day. Medieval Christianity perhaps understood this need to ditch the regular solemnity and sexual decorum and let off steam by sanctioning the Feast of Fools, an annual drunken orgiastic fiesta where anything went. Drinking competitions, praying to vegetables, urinating out of bell towers—and having sex with anyone of any gender. All of which was believed to hold a higher purpose for the clergy at the time: "Wine barrels burst if from time to time we do not open them and let in some air." And man, once aired, can return to serving God with greater zeal. As the philosopher Alain de Botton reflects on the Feast: "We should give chaos pride of place once a year or so, designating occasions on which we can briefly be exempted from the two greatest pressures of secular adult life: having to be rational and having to be faithful."[71]

Perhaps a contemporary incarnation would be to have a National Stray Day. I'm not sure marriage guidance counselors would endorse this. They might be more inclined to point out the result of a major study of couples that showed the key to lasting relationships is being able to generate kindness and generosity. It's not just a matter of being nice to be around, but being generous to the other's ambitions and needs and their desire for space and individuality. The most destructive trait is contempt. Treating your partner with contempt—for example, being mean and critical (Mike's kissing)—can even reduce their ability to fight off cancer.[72] (*Kindness* has now just moved from the flop to a requirement in the first two hole cards.)

Beyond reappraising attitudes to sex, maybe we can also tweak the space in which couples live. We are, after all, tribal animals. The nuclear family ideal, locked away in its own space—further removed as more wealth is accrued—perhaps puts a strain on the relationship. We spend too much time with just each other and also not enough time with other members of our own sex (more to come on that). If chucking it all to move to a commune in a forest isn't your thing, how can we retain our own private spaces while living more of our lives around other people? One way would be to eat together more.[73] For our streets and neighborhoods to be designed so that people could come together at dinnertime rather than secrete themselves away in microunits. Tapping into our tribal roots, having a chance to form wider connections, benefits isolated older people and kids (less "How was your day, dear?" and brooding in front of the TV), and opens up some relationship space that might actually enhance the intimacy: closeness needs its distance. I had a taste of this when I lived on a kibbutz for six months during my preuniversity gap year among a group of 150 or so people living and working together in the baking Israeli desert. It was an intense, idealistic, and extraordinary experience that at times could veer into the cloyingly claustrophobic and where privacy was in scant supply. I soon learned of affairs that even the husbands didn't know about. But my abiding memory was each Friday night when the whole community came together to eat in the dining hall before stepping outside into the communal square to talk, drink, and dance under the laser-sharp stars. It was something atavistically—essentially—human. The polar opposite to binge-watching whatever the latest equivalent to *Breaking Bad* is on your own with a plate balanced on your lap.

What else might we consider in this marital overhaul? Well, if we've really got carte blanche to go for it, I'd say we need to turn down some of the hype around marriage itself. Maybe not go as far as the Mexican lawmakers who proposed two-year renewable marriage contracts.[74] But to take a leaf from that Eastern approach, perhaps we should see a relationship as something that will warm up over time: so, in other words, you find someone you like spending time with, whom you like a lot, when you're well past the 37 percent point so you know that this sort of person doesn't come along every day. Indeed, to take note that the idea of romance in marriage is a relatively new concept that only really started to take root in the West in the eighteenth century—indeed, among the upper classes it was held that excessive passion could result in the birth of unnatural children.[75] Love was almost accidental to marriage,[76] and I daresay in rather short supply in the "wife sales" that persisted in England until at least 1887.[77] Not that we should hold up our repressed Victorian ancestors as relationship role models, but today's expectations of romance—inflated by every rom-com, schmaltzy wedding, and Valentine's assault—are surely too high for our own good. In the Mass Observation reports that peered into the granular lives of ordinary people, among middle-class Americans in the late 1940s/early 1950s, only one in twenty said they were dissatisfied with their marriage. A snapshot today by a US psychologist finds only 30 percent of people are in enduring *happy* marriages.[78] In business, good sense is to underpromise and overdeliver. Our model of relationships damagingly inverts this wisdom.

This isn't to curmudgeonly kill off romance, but rather to let it heat up at an unhurried pace and evolve into something more realistic and ultimately more enduring. So more rom-coms where boy meets girl and ends up quite liking her but not being sure as the credits roll; and more wedding speeches where the groom says, "We seem to have enough physical and cultural commonalities that it bodes well for our long-term compatibility and my chances of embracing the challenge of monogamy. I hope to develop real kindness and generosity toward you over time, and doesn't your middle-finger length look beautiful today." That's one wedding even I'd look forward to.

If all else fails, the *Microtus ochrogaster* might be our salvation. Scientists have found a way of turning the promiscuous meadow vole into a monogamous creature. After an extra vasopressin (V1a) receptor has been inserted into the ventral pallidum region of his brain, the male meadow vole sheds his previous interest in multiple partners and focuses on just one female, even when other females try to tempt him. The colead author of the study believes this extra receptor means that after sex a feel-good chemical is released. "It makes the voles think, 'When I'm with this partner I feel good.' And from then on, they want to spend their time with that particular partner."[79]

How long before a commitment pill at Walgreens?

6

WHEN MORRISSEY CAME FOR TEA

Or we could just go celibate.

Which I pretentiously announced I had become at a party in Manchester one Saturday night in 1989, only to fall off the wagon and make out with a buxom girl from Sale two hours later. I'm not even sure, at thirteen, I knew what the term meant, but Morrissey—for those of you who don't know, the lead singer of the iconic Manchester-based eighties band The Smiths—had declared himself celibate, so that was one of the Moz Commandments to slavishly follow. And follow I did, as I jostled to be chief disciple among the legion of becardiganed Smiths fans mooning around Manchester.

After forensic research, I tracked down Morrissey's own hairdresser at the old Corn Exchange and had the same fingers and scissors perfectly replicate the flattop and quiff, even shaving in a receding hairline. Oscar Wilde poetry was duly procured and the pet hamster named after him. Meat became murder, and Saturdays were spent outside McDonald's handing out those leaflets that featured graphically butchered cows. Vegetarian shoes were even tried, till they were found lacking by a puddle in a Manchester street. Goths were viewed as indie infidels: how could they possibly accept the gospel according to Robert Smith of The Cure?

It was total fandom. Every inch of wall space, which had previously been plastered with Manchester City football—sorry, *soccer*—players, was turned over to The Smiths. A shrine to Morrissey, Marr, et al.

It wouldn't overly tax Dr. Phil to work this one out. "*I lost my stepbrothers, and I still want to feel part of the family*"—perhaps not the most gripping episode, but I'd deduce that's what was going on. I'd put the older brothers in the family my dad had hastily married into onto a pedestal: they were cool, able to get away with more than I could dream of, and happened to be big Smiths fans. Like a fledgling magpie, I picked up their musical taste and, as the marriage went pear-shaped, took the Smiths fandom to another level to retain a connection with them. Whatever pop theories I may retrofit to try to explain to myself why a thirteen-year-old would possibly shave his hairline, The Smiths were also musical manna for a teen whose family life was imploding. To this day, when I listen to the album *The World Won't Listen*, I'm a boy back in bed hearing raised adult voices between the tracks "Asleep" and "Unloveable."

The Smiths T-shirt, cardigan, quiff, murdered-cow leafleting, and Doc Martens were also speedy boarding to a seat on the back of the bus with older boys and the buffet of adolescent vices. So it was that one Saturday, after a day of browsing records in Our Price and smoking on benches on a mundane middle-England main street, we—I, a punk who was a high school senior, his sexy punk girlfriend, and Matt, who was a full foot taller than me—decided to partake in the local sport: some light Morrissey stalking. The Smiths hadn't long split up, but they all lived in the local area. There was an informal arrangement with Morrissey's mom in Hale that you could drop off a record and pick it up signed the next week. Johnny Marr's wife didn't mind if you buzzed on with a T-shirt too. And every now and then, there was the fleeting sighting reported of a majestic quiff peeking out of the top of a white VW Golf convertible.

The four of us trudged up to a house where the latest intel suggested Morrissey was living. There was a Golf outside. As we moped around, wondering whether to ring the bell or not, out sauntered Morrissey. The messiah casually wandered over, chatted with us for most of his Saturday evening, and posed for photos. At the end, I asked if I could do an interview with him for the youth magazine of the Vegetarian Society—who'd been supplying me with the leaflets—and wrote down my phone number. On Monday, I got a call from someone who sounded just like Morrissey but said it wasn't, to arrange to come over the next day. To my flat.

As reasons go for a thirteen-year-old to skip the last lesson of school, "Morrissey is coming round to ours" isn't too shabby. *Sir, I've got one of the world's most influential yet elusive rock stars popping over after school— is it OK to miss math?* And so, that afternoon, math was duly missed, my dad came home from work early poised with his Nikon, and Morrissey rang the buzzer to come up to the flat we lived in. For a man with a reputation for being difficult, he couldn't have been sweeter. He turned up with gifts, braved the shrine of signed multiple images of himself that stared back at him, and patiently sat for two hours at our dining table playfully answering all the daft questions my teen inquisition could muster.

So you think animals should be left alone?
In a little field, by a little tree, with a little bib on—yes! I was very influenced, if it can be said, by Bernard Matthews'* horrible television advertisement in the writing of *Meat Is Murder*. I'm infuriated by TV ads which show chickens laughing as if they can't wait to get in the oven.

How do you feel about wearing leather?
I stopped wearing leather jackets a number of years ago. I do wear leather shoes though, because I can't really see that there is a sensible alternative.

---

*A manufacturer of poultry meat products.

Do you still take royal jelly?
No, it's the property of others, isn't it? The bees work hard for it, and I don't, so now I'm on ginseng, which keeps me as young as I look.

What do you think about people wearing fur?
It's disgusting. They're disgusting. If I'm in a hotel or restaurant and I see someone wearing fur, I ask them to take it out of public view. They usually do. They are deeply offended, wounded, and humiliated, and I think they feel a bit ridiculous, but they still remove it.

Do you think that Thatcher cares about the environment as she now says she does?
No, it was simply seizing the moment to say something that she knew was overdue. Unfortunately, because most newspapers are behind her, they promoted her speech in a very overblown way; but I can't believe at this stage that she cares at all.

Her entire history is one of violence, oppression, and horror. Margaret Thatcher is completely destructive—and she has certainly helped enormously towards the destruction of our planet.

Have you ever made contact with Thatcher?
Well, we had a sauna the other night!—no, I haven't.

Do you shop at supermarkets that don't sell meat?
Well, that's quite hard. I mean, can you name one?

Holland & Barrett.
Well, yes, but I don't think of that as a supermarket, really. I do go to health food shops, but I've also been sighted in Marks & Spencer's: people have got blurred photographs which look like lampshades.

What influence did Meat Is Murder *have on the rest of The Smiths?*
They all became vegetarian.

Why did The Smiths split up?
The Smiths never had a managerial figure, and there were so many horrible business problems that ultimately nobody could stand it. Everybody just ran away, really. I think Johnny [Marr] felt the strain the hardest.

So there's no chance of getting back together?
At the moment, I can't see one, but I'll send you a postcard if I hear of any.

Do you envisage staying in the pop world for a while?
Not massively long term, no.

Couple of years, perhaps?
Oh, all right then, I'll make it one year if you like.

Do you have any advice for people who . . .
. . . who want to give interviews? I'd say don't do it, ha ha!

Having survived the royal jelly and leather shoe interrogation, he politely dodged staying for the soya mince that was en route to the deep fryer pan and slunk off in the VW. A quite amazing experience that only gets more surreal—to me—over time. In my world, it was the equivalent of a Bowie, Lennon, or Dylan in their prime popping over for tea.

Beyond affording schoolboy bragging rights, the episode resonated with a wider ethos that was being inculcated at my high-powered high school: namely, that anything was possible. That no ambition was off-limits. I'd seen that, with a dose of chutzpah, you could get to interview your idol. Simultaneously, the school was purveying the idea that, with application, no job or position in society would be unattainable, an ambition reinforced at pupils' homes by often lower-middle-class parents eager for their offspring to carry on the upward trajectory. It's laudable to fill a kid's head with confidence, to inspire him to perceive no barriers holding him back.

But is there a danger that some schools and parents are overpromising something that adulthood is rarely going to truly deliver? A sense of entitlement that will become a burden once reality makes an appearance, morphing into an internal monologue that bleats you *should* be doing better. Of the many school friends I'm still in touch with, I can't think of any who would say they are truly satisfied with their careers, whatever objective level of success they have attained.

And we grew up in a pre–*X Factor* era. Today, even if you're not lucky enough to have a pushy school or supportive parent, heads are being filled with an entitled assumption that fame and overnight fortune are just a premium-rate text away. Maybe humane teachers should be correctively preaching, "You're not all that, sunshine. And good luck getting a mortgage one day."

It might not have been the full *X Factor*–style slow-motion, piano-laden sequence showing me going back to my hometown in an SUV, but there was a post-Morrissey minor celebrity bump. I was splashed across the local papers, featured in teen girls' magazines, and then called to appear on Saturday morning children's TV to talk about vegetarianism. Sporting a *Meat Is Murder* T-shirt, cardigan, and the freshly defined hairline of a middle-aged man, I appeared on the BBC show *Eggs'N'Baker* with former Eurovision-winning songstress Cheryl Baker, where I cooked a broccoli dish with then boy-band heartthrobs Brother Beyond. Pretty sure that was the moment my career peaked.

I got the media bug. Not just because of the *oh-look-at-me* factor—though I did get one fan letter from a girl—but because I was fascinated by demystifying the mechanics of how it worked. Seeing what was fed into those cathode ray tubes that pumped out the programs I'd spent so much time transfixed by, which had brought me up—the shows that I can still clearly affix to each twist, and home, of childhood.

A couple more children's TV appearances followed. I edited the school newspaper. From fifteen, I spent my Saturdays working at the local radio station, Key 103, as a baby-faced news reporter: heading off on the bus to murder scenes with my tape recorder to ask neighbors if they were shocked that Darren/Wayne/Steve had been killed (they usually were). On my gap year in Israel, I delved into Nazareth to interview Jews and Arabs who'd dared to marry each other—and reported live after a massacre.

The greatest joy came in college, at St. Andrews, when I closed the stodgy newspaper, faced down a mass staff revolt, and launched *The Saint*, which won student newspaper of the year and still exists. Taking a celebratory double-decker bus around the three streets of St. Andrews may have incurred a warning from the constabulary for orchestrating a breach of the peace, but my CV was looking in decidedly good shape, and I earned a place on the hallowed BBC News graduate trainee program. With my history and international relations degree in hand, I'd be stepping into the cathode: off to become a manly TV war reporter.

Morrissey postscript: twenty years after he came over for tea, I was lined up to do another interview with him for the BBC's *Culture Show*. The press release went out that I was remeeting childhood hero Morrissey; it was all set to go. But he then abruptly canceled on the eve of the interview. I later found out that, apparently, Morrissey had googled me and found an article I'd written in my last year at university about giving up vegetarianism by sneaking into McDonald's one day. I wasn't actually angry. There was a reassuring fixity that, out there, the principles I'd signed up for in youth were still solid. And, sometimes, the unself-conscious questions of a thirteen-year-old can't be topped. By the way, Moz, I am virtually vegetarian these days, if you do want to chew the fat.

7
A BAD DAY FOR A MELTDOWN

HOW TO STAY SANE AS A MAN

Of all the days to have a meltdown.

Together with my fellow band of fresh-faced BBC trainees, we were off to meet the corporation's top brass. A chance to go inside the inner sanctum of the world's finest broadcasting organization. Meet the heads of the news programs, sit down with the tea-time anchors we wanted to emulate, gawp at the familiar studios, and then have an audience with the director general (DG) himself.

Pride should have been the predominant emotion. Chests swelling at having started our careers off as trainees on such a privileged trajectory. But, as we were shepherded into an oak-paneled room to meet the most powerful person in broadcasting, my chest was anything but swollen. It was pounding a furious beat. My throat was parched and contracting. My head was spinning into an out-of-body orbit.

Looking down on myself would be to see a young man, hair almost brushed for the occasion, wearing a new gray suit, trying desperately to hold it together while burning up with panic. A brain that had turned to sludgy marshmallow, unable to articulate thoughts, desperate not to be deployed with the impossible task of small talk. Someone who never wanted to be out of a room more, but who was trapped trying to maintain the outward veneer of a graduate thrilled at the onset of his exciting career and by no means having some sort of meltdown in the middle of the DG's office.

It was useful to learn that it's possible to retain an outward veneer of apparent normality even when the mind is going through hell. You never know who—in any given meeting or social event—is really going through what.

That day itself remains a blur. I can't recall with any precision meeting the DG. I do remember muttering to a fellow trainee about not sleeping so well the night before, a bone to throw anyone off the scent. What I really couldn't tell anyone was the reason behind the mental fiasco: Guatemala.

After graduating from St. Andrews six months earlier, with a little time to kill before my traineeship at the BBC began, I'd headed to Central America with the vague notion of picking up a language. After two carefree months exploring Mexico, I met a guy in a hostel who suggested going to Guatemala, so we jumped on a bus, took a boat, and ended up on some island for more of the usual traveler shtick. One night, we had an old-school British pub crawl around whatever bars the island had to offer, and somewhere in among it we smoked some spliff. I'd smoked a little the week or so before and had never experienced anything so potent. I've no idea if it was laced with something or if it was just some sort of Central American superskunk, but I'd lain in bed tripping—vividly floating from my bed up to the ceiling of the rustic hut.

So a few beers, some of that local spliff, and lots of daft war stories to recall over breakfast the next day in a Dunkin' Donuts. Over toast and coffee, I felt something unnerving start to envelop me: panic. Spreading through my body, an alien, gripping anxiety.

Forty-eight hours of drug-fueled panic attacks on a remote island somewhere off Guatemala would struggle to make the full five stars on TripAdvisor. It was about as unpleasant as anything I'd ever experienced: an overwhelming panic far away from anyone or anything familiar. Fearing that I was losing my mind, I jumped on the next boat, plane, and plane to get to my nearest friend—who was up in San Francisco.

With the privilege of hindsight, I realize the best thing I could have done would have been to see a doctor or shrink straightaway who could have told me that I'd just had a bad reaction to the drugs, had a perfectly common panic attack, hadn't caused any lasting damage to my brain chemistry, and should take some sedatives for a while if it flared up again, and generally not worry about it.

Just about the worst thing was not getting that early reassurance to nip my worries in the bud, and then having months to brood on the idea that I'd somehow rewired my brain and would no longer be fit to start my dream job at the BBC. The idle mind is the master of self-sabotage.

By the time I walked into Broadcasting House three months later, I was a tightly wound coil of self-cooked nerves, poised to unravel at the most inopportune moment.

To be fair to the Guatemalan tourist board, I'd had the odd, much more minor "wobble" prior to departing their island in haste. Despite spending my childhood listening to tracks like "Heaven Knows I'm Miserable Now" and "Panic," I wasn't actually an unhappy kid. I can psychoanalyze the ass off my youth to retrospectively spot avoidance mechanisms deployed to overcome various traumas, but I was an inwardly and outwardly happy, confident, popular child. I was sent for a cursory once-over to see a hot trainee counselor after my dad divorced my step-mom; she gave me the all clear, and I spent the session wondering if she might fancy me once my voice broke.

By college, I had begun to experience some passing low moods, especially when I wasn't busy. Negative thoughts—and a clawing lethargy—could creep into the void. Never enough to go back and see or try pulling that counselor, but enough to have put a dent in that all-boys' school all-encompassing arrogance and to belatedly develop a heightened sense of empathy.

Nowadays, intermittent mental wobbles are a mundane fact of life. I can't imagine life without them, who I'd be. They're part of the furniture, nestling alongside overthinking. The shitty yin to whatever positive yang can make you driven, creative, empathetic, a bit different.

With more of that hindsight, I'm not even sure the drugs—which I've not touched since the day I left Guatemala—did more than hasten some of the mind detritus coming up to the surface. As much as I spent years wishing I could have turned back the clock and not left Mexico on a whim, I'm not sure it would really have made that much of a difference over time. It's just part of who I am. Had it not surfaced then, my money would have been on Iraq 2003. During the second Gulf War, I was asked if I wanted to go out to report from Iraq—every reporter's flak-jacketed wet dream and an opportunity the old cocksure me would have jumped at. But to the mystification of colleagues, I politely declined, knowing I'd get PTSD before I even made it out of arrivals at Saddam International.

HOW DOES THIS MAKE YOU FEEL?

I'm not hugely enjoying writing this. It feels exposing to lay your mental health bare. There's no towel to hide behind. It somehow seems like an admission of weakness. And it feels *unmanly*. A little like office tears, it's something that's easier for a woman to be candid about. Elizabeth Gilbert can open *Eat, Pray, Love* by describing her meltdown on the kitchen floor and be met with universal praise, mass empathy, and a sympathetic portrayal by Julia Roberts. As a man, I'm still reticent. It's an underlying sense that you'll be judged, that you've drawn attention to a weakness—a drop of blood in the shark pool of male competition. Perhaps it's only once you have enough credit in the bank—some recognition/objective success—that you feel you can cash in a few chips to reveal your fragilities.

Why, then, hang out the mental laundry? Well, I think there's an urgent need for men to talk about mental health. That might sound like the sort of bromide a generic politician would spout, but on a personal level I can attest to how valuable speaking out can be. When I was first going through a proper moment—doubting that I could ever turn it all around and pull off a career—I drew enormous strength from the rare occasions when I'd read about a well-known man talking about his own mental health issues (whereas, in women's mags you couldn't move for the celebrity confessional).

Take Jeremy Paxman, the former host of the BBC's *Newsnight* and the most feared interviewer in British broadcasting. Somewhere along the line, I'd read that Paxman had depressive tendencies and had banked this. As it happened, after picking myself up from the DG's floor, a couple of years later I went on to win Young Journalist of the Year (beta-blocker for the acceptance speech) and to work on *Newsnight* as a cub reporter. For a young journalist who might be having an off day, it made a genuine difference just to see someone around whose demons hadn't stopped them from reaching the top, demonstrating that having depressive tendencies doesn't define who you are or what you can do.

Over the years, a growing number of successful men have stood up and come "out" and admitted they have faced mental health struggles. In the more confessional culture Stateside, the list of well-known depressive/anxious figures is extensive, including hypermale icons such as Brad Pitt, Jon Bon Jovi, Eminem, and *Mad Men*'s Jon Hamm. In the UK, the stiff upper lip seems to be softening. Well-known figures include sportsmen Freddie Flintoff, Stan Collymore, Ronnie O'Sullivan, Danny Rose; comedians Stephen Fry, Hugh Laurie, John Cleese; musicians Robbie Williams,

Richard Ashcroft; political advisor Alastair Campbell—all hit my radar (and were banked). In Norway, the prime minister Kjell Magne Bondevik took three weeks off from running his country to deal with depression. Sportsmen, politicians, musicians, actors—though, tellingly, not so many top men in business yet, an outpost of cutthroat machismo that needs to join the group hug.

There are rich historical psychological pickings too. With great minds can go a decent dose of angst. John Lennon, Charles Dickens, Franz Kafka, Abraham Lincoln, Isaac Newton, Mark Twain: welcome all to group therapy. And don't forget the man who saved us from the Nazis. In August 1944, the very month that saw D-Day swing the Second World War in the Allies' favor, Winston Churchill mused to his doctor:

> When I was young . . . for two or three years the light faded out of the picture. I did my work. I sat in the House of Commons, but black depression sat on me. It helps me to talk to Clemmie about it. I don't like standing near the edge of a platform when an express train is passing through. I like to stand right back and if possible to get a pillow between me and the train. I don't like to stand by the side of the ship and look down into the water. The second's action would end everything. . . . It helps to write down half a dozen things which are worrying me. Two of them, say, disappear; about two nothing can be done, so it's no use worrying, and two perhaps can be settled.[1]

Nice to know Churchill was an early adopter of CBT list making. Psychological succor also comes from fictional characters. Tony Soprano brooding in therapy and popping happy pills; Larry David trying to sack his shrink after seeing him sport a thong on the beach, or squabbling with Richard Lewis over not sharing a sacred TM mantra—these all normalize the paraphernalia of mental health. Though ending your weekly sessions with a therapist still remains one of the most fraught and farcical experiences known to man: you can't say you're cured (they know you're not), you can't use the line "It's me, not you" (they've known that since the second you met). The only face-saving option is to go AWOL and regard the area surrounding their treatment room as a scene of nuclear fallout never to be breached.

Every time a well-known man confesses to suffering from some sort of mental health struggle, it deepens the well that we can draw inspiration from in the dark times. It chips away at stigma and normalizes what can feel like the most confusing and alienating experience in life. For some men, it will genuinely be easier for them to take the vital step of talking to friends about not feeling well, because of Dwayne Johnson's candor. The awkwardness of first sitting in the therapist's waiting room will feel less alien having seen *The Sopranos* or *Curb Your Enthusiasm*. Bipolar disorder might be less daunting if you've seen *Silver Linings Playbook*.

I know I've drawn tangible comfort over the years from other men's candor, whether that of public figures, close friends, or even fictional characters. But why this wider openness is needed so badly relates to the sheer scale of what we're up against: an awful lot of men out there are having a tough time with their mental health. And we're just not very good at helping ourselves.

FOOTNOTE TO GET US ON *OPRAH*: Interestingly, in an age when the emotional crossover between men and women is greater than ever before, the insight provided by female figures can be harnessed by men too. To my personal mental savings account, I'd also deposit women like Ruby Wax, J. K. Rowling, Lena Dunham, and Oprah herself as sources of inspiration. (Cue whooping.)

MAN DOWN

The statistics paint a tragic picture. Men are three and a half times more likely than women to take their own lives in the United States. Suicide is now the leading cause of death among men aged twenty to forty-nine in England and Wales.[2] Likewise in Australia, and four out of five Canadian suicides are male.[3] This is a global epidemic. Of all the countries with available data, suicide rates among men are three to 7.5 times greater than that of women. Only China and India buck the trend.[4]

An epidemic of men who can no longer bear to go on living.

And an epidemic of men who are battling mental health conditions that can cast such a shadow over life. On paper, more women are diagnosed with depression—some 12 million in the US compared to 6 million men.[5] But the needle is moving the wrong way for men: in the UK, depression rates are rising among men but falling for women. Women are better at recognizing they have a condition, seeking help—being twice as likely to seek treatment if depressed—and pulling back from the ultimate dark act.[6] Men can learn a lot from this readiness to talk, to show vulnerability rather than bottling everything up. Our proud silence is killing us.

The true scale of male depression is unknown. Maybe it's actually on a par with female rates these days? We just don't recognize when we're ill, or if we do suspect something is up, we keep it to ourselves and are less likely to seek help. Canadian mental health workers found "men described their own symptoms of depression without realizing they were depressed. . . . [Men] made no connection between their mental health and physical symptoms, such as headaches, digestive problems, and chronic pain."[7] And, the WHO has found this holds true for men the world over.[8]

The astonishing male suicide rates, and the millions of men who have recognized their depression and sought treatment, are merely the most visible signs of a wider, deeply troubling male malaise.

Throw in: self-medication through alcohol and drug abuse, which men are three times more likely to suffer from; men's self-destructiveness, coupled with anger and violence, which goes some way to explaining why the prison population is 93 percent male in the US[9]; homelessness, a majority male preserve; men not surviving as long as women after their spouse dies[10]; and the fact that 80 percent of children excluded from school for behavioral problems are boys.[11] Again, these are just the tangible barometers. What about the legions of men with eating disorders who go undiagnosed—as many as 25 percent of all cases could be male—as it's not seen as a man thing?[12] Or the dads who have pre- or postnatal depression—who even knew *that* existed?[13] The 30 million–plus American men whose self-esteem might be shaky after being diagnosed with clinical obesity? Those overworking to blot out the angst? And the countless number of men who are going through the motions of life but with that sinking feeling *This is as good as it'll get*. Chewing life without tasting it. Perfunctory hunter-gathering.

If one of the biggest factors holding men back from confronting or talking about their mental health is that fear of being judged—to be seen as *other* or somehow less manly—then take comfort in the sheer number of men who definitely won't be judging you but will in fact know where you're coming from. Tot up all the men who contribute to these cheery statistics and percentages—not to mention the guys who helped make Prozac and its fellow happy pills the most commonly prescribed drugs in the US in the previous decade—and we're not dealing with something that's niche. If you're prone to mental health angst, consider yourself in the mainstream. And in some pretty reputable—current and historical—company. Normal serotonin levels are just so passé.

Men might be too proud, or unaware of symptoms, to recognize that there could be something mentally amiss. As I discovered in Guatemala, it can be so hard to know what's going on other than having a terrifying sense of losing your mind. It's also difficult, though, to find the right language to talk about mental health, to tell people what it is you're feeling. And in a way that doesn't feel emasculating.

I'm lucky enough to have some close friends who are also prone to episodes (try working in the media and not being); we've developed a shortcut emotion-free terminology that seems to work. In case it's vaguely useful to share, here it is:

Mental cold: low-level depression/angst, feeling a bit shitty, sleep not great, struggling to motivate, patchy libido, fairly antisocial

Mental flu: more pronounced and debilitating. Feeling listless, really not like yourself, spaced out at times, widespread negativity, zero libido and sociability, disturbed sleep; root causes need addressing

Mental pneumonia: a real struggle to get through the day, mind feels like it's turned to sludge; serious bout of illness, demands proper attention, mercifully rare

Hopefully, the negative patches tend to be fleeting or intermittent for many, rather than ongoing. Mental wobbles are like the weather. There are times when a bad front will blow in; you acknowledge it's going to be unpleasant for a while, but it will go away.

In an unpredictable climate, the symptoms can mix and match without any obvious logic. Stress/anxiety can descend while you're seemingly feeling in a good mood. Last week, for a couple of days, I felt a physical stress in my body—a tenseness that was uncomfortable at times, but plow-on-through-able. I've no idea what the trigger was. But something in how my mind saw the world set off stress hormones. We are wired to release cortisol and epinephrine when our lives are in danger: when that lion pops up on the savannah, when a house catches fire. Hormones that temporarily flood the body to raise alertness and provide a stash of get-away glucose. Yet, my fight-or-flight mechanisms had been triggered by . . . what? Probably some underlying stress about not knowing what my next big work project was going to be—the contemporary equivalent of looking around the prairie and having no idea where the next kill is coming from. And those hardcore hormones that are supposed to be released in short bursts kept seeping out for days. I don't dare look up the side effects of stress, but I'm pretty sure they don't tend to include a regrowth of hairline and an impromptu six-pack.

WORK. IT FUCKS YOU UP

Problems are so much easier when you can find someone else to blame. The poet Philip Larkin may have pinpointed mothers and fathers as the source of fuckuppery, but who else can we blame for this widespread male malaise?

It's hard not to look past work as the obvious prime suspect: the symbiotic link between a man's self-worth/identity and his primordial breadwinning. Take the recent recession. Job security collapses, and there's a spike in male suicide rates: an estimated 10,000 additional deaths in North America and Europe attributed to the economic downturn.[14] In the UK, that fatal surge was especially discernible among middle-aged men: the suicide rate increased by 11 percent for men in their forties and early fifties, the guys whose raison d'être at home and in society is often so toxically tied to what they do for a living.[15] The immediate cause and effect is just that demonstrable. As one psychologist recalls:

I assessed a married father who found himself on a station platform contemplating a violent suicide after his IT role was relocated abroad. Fortunately, he soon found alternative employment as a door-to-door salesman and, miraculously, his depression and suicidal ideation disappeared.[16]

With the blessing of perspective, it seems crazy. That a living organism, the product of 360 million years of evolution from amphibian to humanoid—or, if you prefer, a life created by an all-loving God—born from the most eager of 60 million sperm, should extinguish itself because of an overseas IT relocation. Crazy, yet wretchedly real. We are so zoomed in on our lives; and when a lens is at full zoom, the slightest movement feels like a massive disruption.

Nor is this correlation between a man's work and his mental well-being any sort of modern phenomenon. It's sometimes hard for us to imagine that men living in entirely different eras could have had the same feelings or thought processes as we do—much as we might find it hard to believe that an old person was ever capable of developing a crush. But just as man's body has barely changed for thousands of years, so his need to "do" has been all too familiar over the centuries.

After just a week of unemployment, a young American man in 1844 whined to his girlfriend about the "painful vacancy in my mind," complaining that "the 'Blues' seem to be already gathering around me."[17] Try being freelance, pal.

His work angst was far from isolated. The challenges of industrialization, with its changes to job security and the way of working, led to the diagnosis of a new male-centric disease in 1869 by one Dr. George Beard: *neurasthenia*, or "brain sprain." Men across the northern United States were felled by this new condition, which brought about fatigue, depression, indigestion, increased drinking, and headaches. It reached near epidemic proportions among middle-aged men, even striking down future presidents Theodore Roosevelt and Woodrow Wilson.[18] "Brain sprain" was seen as a disease of the "fast life" in modern cities; the result of cutting-edge technologies like steam power, the telegraph, and regular newspapers.[19] Doctors at the time believed the human body had a finite amount of energy, and all this new "brain work" of the middle class was dangerously draining men's systems.

Interestingly, there wasn't any stigma attached to suffering from neurasthenia, as the unimpeded progress of Wilson and Roosevelt showed. In fact, the condition was actually seen as a sign of progress: that society was now moving at a faster pace, even outstripping man's physical abilities to keep up.[20] Imagine if such an attitude could be adopted today? If those suffering from mental illness—today's all-too-familiar version of "brain sprain"—could be applauded for being at the vanguard of society's progress?

Given those finite energy reserves, the cure for men was to send them off to recuperate in a suitably macho environment. They were dispatched to dude ranches to recharge their energy and masculinity, resting their minds under cowboy hats.[21]

Women at the time suffering from nervous conditions were not prescribed an invigorating dose of the Wild West. They were ordered to retreat to total domesticity: one young woman was told to stay at home, lie down after each meal for an hour, and "never touch a pen, brush, or pencil as long as you live."[22] With women having been dismissed as "hysterical" for 4,000 years,* and with thousands killed for being witches—the treatment of women's mental health hasn't been a high point in the history of civilization.[23]

The times when I've been in most need of donning chaps and a Stetson have more often than not been as a result of work. The biggest factor affecting my happiness, sociability, sleep, energy, and even libido is how work happens to be going. A busy and productive me is pretty darn robust. Throw in some meaning and status and we're really cooking. I know that

---

*The word *hysteria* derives from the Greek word for "uterus." Ancient Greek medicine had a concept of "hysterical suffocation," with the symptoms being attributed to a flaw in the uterus.

reflects terribly on my psyche and work-life balance—and I resent work's ability to roam and pillage so freely in my mind, not to mention its weird access to the secret tear duct codes, but there is a certain sort of logic to it.

Work underpins not just how I spend my days and how much I earn; it is the shortcut for identity and social ranking (*"So, what do you do?"*); the adult incarnation of external validation that began when grading started at age four at primary school; and, beyond family, it's the most obvious way to seek some sort of meaning in life. "Meaning," that nebulous concept, which strangely seems to be what it's all about: what will actually pass the litmus test of feeling worthwhile as you're about to kick the bucket. And, since time immemorial, man's meaning has come from *doing*.

This work dominance clearly isn't healthy. Psychologists talk about life as a stool, where it's key to have as many robust legs as possible. So you'll still be standing strong when the work leg is shaky. Or if disaster strikes another leg—say, family—then you're not going to collapse. Indeed, an underlying theme of this book is exploring the different legs that support men today: seeing how well suited they are to weather modern life and asking what could make us more robust, especially when you factor in how, for better or worse, we've lived through history and how we might have been designed to live. There's more than one way to skin this cat of life.

MODERN LIFE VS. MAN

As dominant as work may be for some, if not many, the psychological plight of modern men can't be pinned on just it (and if we do have an inbuilt need to be productive—to *do*—then there are other ways to achieve this beyond the narrow confines of work, which we'll look at in the next chapter). Relationships, with that potential to add or knock off years from your life expectancy, have a big role in psychological well-being. Physical health too. Genetic disposition also plays a part in whether you're a miserable sod or not or if you might be vulnerable only in certain situations. Likewise, I wonder whether some people have a natural quota for worrying—and something always has to fill the vacuum. If so, then at least you know that whatever happens to be that night's anxiety might only be keeping the seat warm till a legitimate concern comes along and should be given the credence of a Comical Ali pronouncement. (During a dose of mind-addling insomnia, I once tried imagining Saddam Hussein's former spokesman—he who denied the invasion as the tanks could be heard behind him—at the lectern, delivering a press conference vocalizing whatever pointless thought was keeping me up. It did wonders to debunk the nocturnal hold of sleeplessness.)

But whatever the genes, however the career and family are going, there is something about modern life that makes it hard for men to walk around in a state of blissful contentment, air-punching at what a great day they're having. All too common is the man who's carrying around unidentified bottled-up angst, with the threat of depression, divorce, or self-destructive behavior lurking below the surface.

If Victorian men were wilting under the pressure of steam-powered trains, how would they fare penned up in the subway at rush hour? If electronic telegraphs can help sprain the brains of the twenty-sixth and twenty-eighth presidents of the United States, what's it doing to us mere mortals to be plugged into a mobile-telegraph device for all waking hours (and nocturnal pee trips)? They may have hailed the progress of society's advance, but has it now turned a revolution too far?

Has today's way of living—this ceaseless intrusion, matched by a bewildering array of choice, information, and decisions—overevolved beyond what's actually good for men (and women)?

Compare my existential things-to-do list to what my great-grandfather may have mentally scribbled on his midnineteenth-century version of the sticky note.

To do (today):

1. Find someone to spend the rest of my life with who is kind (oh, yes), driven but not narcissistic, who will remain sexy and attractive past the initial lust phase, with nice nurturing instincts, who wouldn't be bad to grow old with, not anti-Semitic, small bum, around the ideal age range, living within about fifteen miles of me on this vast planet—who will happen to put up with me.

2. Urgently address expectations re the above or end up a lonely old man waiting for the unicorn to appear.

3. Achieve enough work success to be free to make the documentaries I care about, make a real difference to people's lives and perceptions, and retire in thirty years with a BBC2 night heralding my peerless creativity rather than just petering out in a sad trail of unrequited pitching e-mails.

4. Earn enough money to not have to stress about it, shop at Whole Foods without guilt, and, if 1) comes to fruition, afford a house that's near a subway station but not in a depressingly bland suburb, bring up kids where Dad isn't stressed about money, and be able to afford nice family vacations and private school if the local comp is a bit too rough.

5. Be a good/better son, brother, uncle, more available friend.

6. Consume less dairy, exercise more, get out of bed earlier.

7. Get a dog (nonshedding).

8. Be able to look back at life and say, "That was all right; I gave it my best shot."

I'd like to think that my ancestor had more pressing matters than cosmic ordering an Italian greyhound. His list might have extended to:

To do (*c.* 1850):

1. Marry one of the two single women in the village, ideally the less hairy one if the community decides this on my behalf.
2. Rear and kill enough animals to be able to feed the family and sell a few to trade for shoes.
3. Hope bubonic plague doesn't jump over from Asia.
4. Pile whole family on a boat to escape marauding Russians intent on wiping out the entire village in a pogrom.
5. Keep God happy.

How he would marvel at—or mock—the concerns that fill our heads today. The rampant entitlement and unchecked expectations.

NOT-SO-GREAT EXPECTATIONS

Expectations. So key to how satisfied we feel, as we saw not only in dating and relationships but also across the board. When not comparing life to household furniture, psychologists talk about the gap between our expectations and reality as utterly key. The narrower the gap, the greater the chances of being content. When my great-grandfather lived in a rural village in Russia, his expectations for what life had to offer—what would be a measure of success—would be set by a fairly limited range of factors: the couple of hundred people he might meet throughout his lifetime, the villages he might traverse over a limited number of miles, his rudimentary education, the stories he would have heard that had been passed down through generations, the religious sermons and whatever reading matter might have been around.

Imagine what your expectations—for life, work, love, happiness—would be if you had never seen a film, read a lifestyle magazine, been harangued by advertising, or traveled far and wide, seeing how thousands of other people live. Or been educated to believe that you can be whatever you want to be in life, or lived in a society that worships in the creed that everything is possible.

Our expectations are absurdly, impossibly high. And the nature of the society means they are constantly moving. Like a mouse being tormented by a piece of cheese on a string, our desires get pulled away just as we think we're about to pounce on them once and for all. And we never learn. If I can just get to *that* promotion, reach *that* salary, move to *that* house with *that* woman/man, then I'll definitely be truly happy. No matter the evidence to the contrary: the film stars who have it all yet populate rehab clinics, the lottery winners who wish they'd never bought the ticket, the accident victims whose lives were thrown off designated course yet bounce back as happy as before, the smiley "poor" people we pass in India who haven't got a pot to piss in but (to our patronizing confusion) seem far happier than anyone in the office; no matter, we keep chasing the cheese.

And men aren't just chasing the astronomic expectations that come with advanced capitalism. Somewhere between clearing his in-box, marrying by about thirty, procreating by thirty-five, hitting work seniority by forty-five, and retiring with comfort at sixty-five or so, a man has a whole other set of age-old cultural expectations that stubbornly persist. He is still expected to "be a man"—whatever that means. An imprecise demand that invokes heroism, valor, strength, and independence. A cultural hand-me-down from generations of forefathers that seems a little ill-fitting for today. Strength, heroism, and a hint of aggression aren't exactly the values celebrated in offices and homes across the land; in fact, they are more likely to be an impediment to work success. Yet it's the timeless *tough* incarnation of man that still dominates the Hollywood ideal beamed back at us, still permeates the language used to bring up boys (*be strong, don't cry, man up, don't be such a girl*), and no doubt still has a restless place in our psyche. Raised on a diet of Bond and Bourne

112

and then set loose to hunt in a world of PowerPoint and 360-degree evaluations.

* * *

If we're still playing the role of aggrieved bear looking for someone to blame—*Who's been elevating my expectations?*—then it's none of the usual societal scapegoats. No illegal immigrants, Jews, blacks, Mexicans, gays, Gypsies, or Goldilocks. The real culprit is wafting nonchalantly in the wind: wheat.

As Yuval Noah Harari points out in *Sapiens*, wheat has a lot to answer for: "How did wheat convince *Homo sapiens* to exchange a rather good life for a more miserable existence?"[24] Before the agricultural revolution took root 12,000 years ago or so, we were running around without expectations. Life was hand to mouth. Get up, roam, hunt, build fire, eat, sleep. Repeat. But then we thought we could have a better life if we could drop all that roaming and hunting by growing crops and settling in one place. Food on tap. But with it came the need to start planning ahead—to build expectations around future yields, to look back at what worked with past crops. And with that, the birth of that crippling human condition "if only." *If only* I could have *that* piece of land, a bit more water, a sacrifice to make the wheat-god happy—*then* I'd have crops to die for. The start of cheese-chasing.

And the end of being "present"—the holy grail of the modern mindfulness movement: living in the here and now rather than negatively getting caught up in thought loops reliving the past or preliving what the future will be. That pure sense of your mind totally focused on the job at hand. Which is exactly where we were before wheat cropped up. A hunter-gathering forefather wouldn't have woken up in the middle of the night to worry about whether the wildebeest kill last month was going to represent the peak of his killing career or how life would be so much better if only he could get a cave extension.

In the end, the allure of cereal grains was just too much for man. Though let's not get all Luddite and bemoan the whole sweep of progress over the last dozen millennia. I daresay being a Stone Age man with a toothache can't have been much fun. And the infant mortality rates that ravaged even developed societies until comparatively recently must have brought a terrible darkness to life. But progress isn't, of course, uniformly positive.

Today, this fusion of work insecurity with sky-high expectations about how we should be living, the sheer pace of the modern world, the ever-present technological intrusion, and those anachronistic yet stubborn demands to "be a man" all converge to make life for men complicated at best. Challenging for many. And for a serious number of boys and men, a world prone to self-destructive behavior and mental illness.

PRESCRIPTION

What to do, other than boycott Shredded Wheat?

Suffering is naturally part of the human condition. Buddha and Nietzsche have nailed that. To know pleasure we have to experience pain, and so forth. And we might willingly accept that a certain amount of suffering is part of the bargain for chasing the dreams we have set ourselves or for the lives we want to live. I might have better mental health if I'd chosen to stay in local news, but it's a trade-off I've made with my eyes open to have the chance of reaching greater heights and more "meaning." (Would an Emmy be worth a breakdown and a week at The Meadows? What's the exchange rate?) Just as the Victorians saw "brain sprain" as a sign of progress, we might sacrifice some personal sanity for our own advancement. At some point, we hopefully come to realize the cheese isn't worth it.

Some suffering is inevitable—and some willingly tolerated—but the sheer scale demands action. When the biggest killer of young men isn't cars or illness but themselves, then it should be a political priority. Even from a cold financial perspective, major depressive disorder alone comes at a huge economic cost—an estimated $444 billion a year in the US[25]; in Canada, the impact of mental health is $50 billion a year (nearly 3 percent of its GDP).[26] Globally, it's estimated to reach a whopping $6 trillion by 2030.[27] Some 20 percent of the working-age population within the OECD are suffering from a mental disorder.[28] People across the world are in distress and not reaching their full economic potential. Yet none of the UN's new Sustainable Development Goals even refer to mental health (nor do boys and men even get a mention).[29] It should be right up there in the UN's priorities.

On a domestic level, why not have a cabinet-level secretary for mental health? Someone to specifically champion rolling out effective therapies, drive drugs research, run educational programs so as to catch conditions early among schoolchildren, campaign to tackle stigma, fight cutbacks—and signal that these are just other illnesses, every bit as much as a broken bone or heart condition. Agriculture has its own cabinet secretary—yet contributes just 1 percent of the nation's GDP.[30] Why not have a Secretary of Mental Well-being who could focus on the 3–4 percent of GDP lost to mental illness? Right up there in our new secretary's in-tray would be finding what works for men, harnessing the very best thinking to get us talking and treated.

It's also clearly in the interest of big companies to improve the mental health of their employees—but remarkably, for something with obvious financial gain, there's a patchy approach. Most businesses don't have mental health policies in place, and, not surprisingly, the majority of people affected by such a condition don't feel secure in revealing it to their employers.[31] Work is the biggest source of stress in people's lives, outstripping debt, poor health, and relationships.[32] Yet too many companies do nothing. It's bonkers, immoral, and bad business.

The media holds real sway in changing preconceptions—and nowadays seems to be doing a lot better at creating sympathetic characters in storylines (from soaps to high-end drama), running destigmatizing documentaries, and not reveling in the "mental" headlines when someone suffers a breakdown. Governments, media, and companies can absolutely play their part, but in the end, an awful lot will come down to men's individual choices. The pressures we face, from mass media–fueled hopes to technological intrusion, aren't going away. What will make the difference is how we face down those pressures, keep the stool steady, and—if susceptible to problems—have therapies at hand that do the job.

One way of doing this is by drawing on a mixture of Eastern and Western therapeutic wisdom. The Western approach seems principally focused on pills and talking therapy. Therapy really is horses for courses. I personally prefer a spot of limited, targeted CBT rather than the open-ended analysis and ruminations over childhood. But I have friends who swear by the full-on Freudian-style of lifting of the hood. Either way, it's healthy to have someone to talk to about absolutely anything without being judged, who can spot your repeat patterns and will always be up for another fifty minutes of self-consumed tedium.

As for the alternative approach, some of the most powerful treatments I have personally experienced stem from the East.

What works?

Acupuncture. I am generally needle averse and have manfully fainted during two blood tests, but I have had remarkable results with acupuncture. You can feel almost "reset" after a session, with your energy and mood pushed back in a better direction. And it seems to be an alternative therapy that stands up to scientific scrutiny: studies have found it can help alleviate depression/anxiety, potentially with the same sort of potency as Prozac.[33] Memo to Secretary . . .

Meditation. An intimidating doctor barked at me to go and learn Transcendental Meditation (TM) years ago. Too scared to argue, I duly trotted off to learn TM over a couple of evenings. This was the meditation the Beatles had embraced in the late sixties, so it felt role model–normalized. During their six or so weeks with the Maharishi, they penned thirty or more songs, including most of the White Album. To be fair, I came back from my couple of evenings in Bristol in the late nineties with some epic local-news ideas. TM has been a godsend at times. Twenty minutes of trying to internally repeat the mantra you're given might not sound like much, but afterward it can feel as if you've emerged from a deep sleep—and can profoundly switch off stress/anxiety. In my local-news days, I used to sometimes slip off to the lavatory to meditate: not so Zen when the next-door cubicle is in full swing. (Companies: please provide meditation areas at work. Your staff will be less stressed and more productive and creative.) Exponents—from Clint Eastwood to filmmaker David Lynch, who funds TM courses for at-risk kids—point out the studies showing how repeated practice can lower blood pressure, slow down aging, and even start to bring about neurological changes in the "worrying" parts of the brain. I'm sure it can—and the perennial New Year's resolution is to TM more.

Mindfulness. With its meditations, breathing exercises, and CBT-fueled philosophy designed to keep us present, this is another powerful tool I've found, especially when I'm more in the mood for a guided meditation to calm the mental chatter or wanting to draw on the strange intensity of a group of people meditating together.

Yoga. Another mood game changer. The combination of breathing and an animalesque physical absorption in stretching, twisting, and sweating. The physical seems to be a core factor in supporting the mental, whether through yoga, martial arts, or more vigorous exercise. Perversely, when depressed, people can find going to the gym or a yoga class can be an Everest-like challenge. A friend with a cattle prod helps.

I tend to think, in dark times: chuck the kitchen sink at it and see what works. Take the best the West has to offer and vacuum up the thousands of years of wisdom distilled in the East. Whatever gets you through the night.

I'M AFRAID OUR TIME IS UP

Even now, I find myself falling into the trap of equating male physical appearance with mental robustness. I was recently talking to a guy who was tall, good-looking, well-built, with tattooed muscled arms, and a buzz cut. As he described the time when he was stricken by panic attacks on the way to work, I caught myself wondering, *How can he have panic attacks?* An absurd judgment from someone who does know better, yet the thought briefly crept into my mind. There are countless men walking around who, whatever their appearance happens to be, are suffering inside, some so profoundly that life can become wretched.

Ultimately, life is about striving for the right abundance of three chemicals in the brain: serotonin, oxytocin, and dopamine.[34] The alchemy for happiness. For a man these days, it's tough to get all three flowing. At a time when the idea of what it is to be a man has never been less anchored, we are beset by a range of choices and hopes that would confound our ancestors. There are so many different ways to live life; is the one that you or I am sticking to right now really the best one for us or something that we've just fallen into? If we take a step back from the day-to-day, put aside the norms we take for granted, and are honest about our deepest needs, what would really get those three chemicals kicking?

It's a huge question that encompasses every aspect of life. But while we as mere individuals with rent and mortgages to pay are trying to figure this out, politicians, businesses, and the media should be doing more to take the edges off modern life. Men, ourselves, need to take some responsibility too for smashing whatever residual stigma is out there holding us back from admitting we're not feeling great. We've just got to try talking more. Every man who puts his hand up to admit that he's having a tough time makes it easier for the next guy to say, "I'm not feeling well—but I'm still a man." And any guy who still has the gall to judge another for mental illness should be put in the ring with a depressed Tyson Fury.

8
HOW WAS YOUR DAY, DEAR?

HOW TO SURVIVE THE OFFICE
(AND AVOID GOING ON A SHOOTING SPREE)

Average working week for hunter-gatherer 0.2 million years ago: thirty-five hours
Average working week for American man today: forty-one hours[1]
Average working week for Frenchman today: thirty-five hours (minus strikes)

Let's try to conceive of the most ill-suited way for a man to spend the majority of his waking hours.

- Start by boxing him inside a hermetically sealed building, away from nature, with no fresh air, and immune to the changing of the seasons that have been the centerpiece of life and even worshipped for the last 12,000 years.
- Make him sit down all day, contrary to the active lifestyle adopted by every form of human who has lived since

diverging from chimps six million years ago. Watch as the hunter-gatherer metabolism—now faced with 37 percent of men spending less than thirty minutes of their entire working day on their feet—slows down, sending sugar levels, blood pressure, and fat breakdown haywire.[2]

- Deny his natural sociable instincts. Make him eat half or so of his lunches at his desk, alone. Make him interface with technology, not people, all day. Push this technological domination so far that it creates new conditions, like carpal tunnel syndrome and other repetitive strain injuries (RSIs), caused by the body moving in ways it's not meant to.

- Constantly reinforce his sense of hierarchical position by keeping in the same space—or close by—those who wield direct power over what his annual allocation of resources and level of status will be. This in-your-face hierarchy will play havoc with his serotonin, the neurotransmitter that is key to depression and well-being. The higher a vervet monkey rises up the pack, the greater his serotonin level: low status equals low serotonin.[3] More dominant monkeys also have higher testosterone levels.[4]

- Allow hugely destructive stress hormones to build up over time—sometimes years, exacerbated by this status jostling—rather than to fire up and dissipate in short bursts as the body intends. Deny any physical exertion that might break down this buildup of stress. As a result of this stress, sleep, appetite, relationships, and mental and physical health will be affected. Sick leave will be 62 percent higher in open-plan offices, but hey, cram him in.[5]

- Guarantee that there is enough constant background distraction—especially being able to monitor what his potential rivals are up to—to make total concentration near

121

impossible, such that even his ability to do basic math will be affected.[6] The distraction will ensure that he's never able to reach that mindful state of being totally absorbed in the task in hand.

- Divorce his work from any tangible productivity. There is rarely to be a finished product, with tasks often open-ended.

- Overwhelmingly link his whole sense of identity and esteem to what goes on in this sealed space.

- Ensure that any display of traditional male values that have been lauded for centuries—such as aggression, conflict, a maverick stance, or hypercompetitiveness—will be heavily frowned upon and could lead to the expulsion from the space. Instead, the traditionally female emphasis on consensual decision making will be dominant. Men, apart from the knuckle-dragging Wall Street or Square Mile species, will have to bend to fit this way of the world.

- Replace the wider sense of tribe, which has been integral throughout man's existence, with a quasi community populated by the other random people who happen to occupy this building. However, the bonds in this surrogate community are not to be built on shared genes, history, or concerns, and a man can be dismissed from this new tribe by a piece of paper giving him a perfunctory period of notice.

- Co-opt the sixteenth-century navy practice of hot bedding—crew members on different shifts sharing one bunk—to hot desking, ensuring that a man won't have his own piece of office territory. Something that would drive your pet dog nuts.

Yet around 70 percent of us trudge across town each day to be boxed into these work pens that sap our serotonin, testosterone, productivity, and identity. And that reward us with bad backs, diabetes, and "pink noise" pumped in so that we won't feel too self-conscious to actually speak out loud. At least at the Google office in Zurich there's a slide between floors, to ensure you really don't have to spend any time on those awkward toe-studded growths on the end of your legs.

Taming man, turning him into a submissive corporate creature, hasn't come easily. The macho characteristics that were ideal for empire- and nation-building needed to be knocked out of him when it came to growing twentieth-century companies. Those hardy manly values of rivalry and fighting that were all the rage while settling frontiers and "taming" the natives.[7]

Some foresaw the writing on the (cave) wall for men. A crisis of masculinity was declared more than a hundred years ago, with workplaces, homes, and even cities themselves seen as dangerously feminizing influences on men. "The masculine tone is passing out of the world; it's a feminine, a nervous, hysterical, canting age," declares a Civil War veteran in Henry James's 1886 novel, *The Bostonians*. From the 1920s, that writing had moved from wall to flip chart, as droves of men were sent off to learn "people skills." While foremen and middle managers were sent to "retraining sessions"—to be less male—salesmen were shipped off to Dale Carnegie classes to learn how to win friends and influence people and to internalize the injunction that "If You Want to Gather Honey, Don't Kick Over the Beehive."[8]

Amid the 360-degree evaluations, having to nip outside to make a phone call, furtive Facebooking, and staring ever-so-intently at the screen whenever a boss passes within ten feet, did anyone get the memo: *Was It All Worth It?*

HANDY MAN

The last hundred years represent 0.05 percent of our 200,000 years on earth as *Homo sapiens*. For the overwhelming majority of that time—and the 2 million years before that in our *Homo erectus* guise—careers fairs would have been limited occasions. The only stall would have been offering a vocation in foraging, though some tribes may have gone with a "hunter-gathering" rebranding (same old foraging dressed up in new loincloths). The job spec wouldn't have been too bad:

- Thirty-five-hour working week
- Hunting one day out of three
- Gathering for three to six hours a day
- Varied and nutritious diet (all organic)
- Few infectious diseases; excellent potential to exercise and tone muscle
- On-the-job training in knife-making, bear-trapping, botany, and weather forecasting[9]
- Must like dogs
- Foraging is an equal opportunity employer: men and women are treated equally

"On the whole, foragers seemed to have enjoyed a more comfortable and rewarding lifestyle than most of the peasants, shepherds, laborers, and office clerks who followed in their footsteps," notes Yuval Harari.[10]

Wheat came along and screwed us. (Why do breakfast cereals have it in for us? If it's not Shredded Wheat ruining our foraging fun, it's Corn Flakes trying to clamp anti-erection devices on our cocks.) We became tied to the land and at the whim of drought and famine and prone to new diseases; our brain sizes shrunk. Expectations and what-ifs took hold in that smaller gray matter, and sexism was born. Before this, women had enjoyed substantial authority and power in foraging society, with the nuts, seeds, and berries they gathered often providing more of the calorific intake than the animals that men spent their time talking about hunting.[11]

The farming life, which kicked in 10,000–12,000 years ago, did at least allow men to spend their days outside, doing something physically productive, perhaps working as their own bosses, often toiling alongside their sons. The sense of working with a physical skill, and having autonomy over what you did, persisted until the nineteenth century. At the time of the Civil War, in the 1860s, nine out of ten men were small farmers, artisans, or shopkeepers.[12] A way of life railroaded by industrialization. An exodus of men from farms to factories, via brain sprain, to paper-pushing amid pink noise.

It's easy to overromanticize manual labor and blot out the hours of total clock-watching tedium. When I look back on the six months I spent picking and packing melons in the Negev desert when I was eighteen, I tend to remember walking to work as the sun rose over the Jordanian mountains. The sense of achievement when all the day's melons were packed, the pallets wrapped and loaded onto trucks. The satisfying physical exhaustion at the end of the day—so different from a mental tiredness from office work—followed by uninterrupted sleep. The Friday nights when everyone would go hedonistically bonkers, drink the cheapest Russian vodka, dance in a bomb shelter, and wake up in any number of beds. Once with two new front teeth. A nice adventure for a young, privileged man to have before heading off to a posh university and hardly representative of the lifestyle endured by the thousands of Latin Americans and Eastern Europeans who pick the fruit and veggies in the US and UK, which the Americans and Brits won't stoop to do.

On the kibbutz, there was a pride too, a wider sense of purpose. We weren't just picking melons—we were part of a community that, in the

Israeli desert, was rooted in an egalitarianism that saw everyone paid the same wage no matter what job they did, where lunches were communal, and everyone came together for that Friday night of breaking bread.

Perhaps it was some of that same wider belonging and purpose that led, by 1900, to some 95 percent of all miners' sons following their fathers into the pits.[13] Despite the backbreaking work and hazardous conditions, and with an acknowledgment that there was little other work available, there's a pride that runs through mining: to do what your dad is doing, to be keeping the country running, and to be facing down the daily fear of not knowing if you'll be coming out of the pit with your head in one piece that day. From Wales to Kentucky, miners have taken to song and poetry to express a fatalistic, grittily romantic view of their lives: filled with exhortations for sons to choose a different path, honoring those who have died underground, yet infused with pride—maybe akin to the verse of soldiers.

> Each dawn as we rise, Lord, we know all too well,
> We face only one thing—A pit filled with hell.
>
> To scratch out a living The best that we can,
> But deep in the heart, Lies the soul of a man.[14]

I'm not sure working in an accounting firm has produced quite the same canon of poetry, song, or brass-band brotherhood. Though, let's not be too hasty in dismissing this corporate anthem.

> KPMG,
> We're strong as can be,
> A dream of power and energy.
> We go for the goal,
> Together we hold
> On to our vision of global strategy . . .[15]

And breathe.

Manual work allied to a wider purpose and community can be an entirely different proposition from laboring just to scrape together a living. As can having a skill. Tradesmen are, apparently, twice as likely to be "extremely happy" in their jobs compared to white-collar workers.[16] Men do love to master a skill. As I sit here, a builder clanging away on a nearby house is belting out "Hit Me Baby One More Time"—for the third time today. I can't recall the last time anyone in a newsroom broke out into spontaneous song. My friend John, a corporate lawyer working beside me today, says he has yet to see a partner burst into Britney. But maybe that's because construction scores right near the top of the happiest occupations, while the media and law are down there scraping the misery barrel with real estate agency.

Without hauling him off the scaffolding for an interrogation, I'd guess the singing builder takes pleasure from seeing a finished product as a result of his labors, from working up a sweat, having skills that others don't, being able to move around firms easily if he doesn't like who he works with, having the potential to be his own boss, and not having hitched his identity since childhood to being a builder. Or maybe he'll be on *The Voice Mexico* next week, desperate to get that big break away from construction surveys about how happy he should be.

The most dispiriting "job" I ever did was technically "semiskilled." When I was a local news reporter and needed to get access to film the dilapidated state that the billion-dollar-plus Millennium Dome project had fallen into, I figured the only way in was to become a security guard. So off I went to train as a security guard. As I sat in a dire function room in a dire hotel near Heathrow for a week, the other guys on the course— middle-aged men and the odd school leaver—all perked up when we were given the corporate spiel about how this could be the start of a dynamic, opportunity-rich career. When we all regrouped after spending a few days at our locations, I'd never felt a room with more air sucked out of it.

Dynamic career, my ass. We'd had a vision of the zombie automata that Henry Ford had told his engineers to create a century before, where human thought was to be eliminated as inefficient.[17] When I patrolled the Dome, I had no discretion over which route to even walk around a room; I had to follow a set path, swiping my pass at fixed stations to prove that I'd adhered to this order. It was soul-destroying work. To be sitting alone in a three-foot-square cubicle for ten hours where your only responsibility was to push a barrier-raising button whenever a car happened to approach. When I did this as a shadow duty, to learn the ropes from another guard as we settled down for our ten hours of cubicle time together, he pulled out a copy of *The Watchtower* and asked if I believed in Jehovah. Conversion never ensued, nor did detection—though it was bloody close when "Officer Samuels" was radioed in to change into a new uniform in the boss's office while I had a secret camera strapped to my back. (I used the same choreography that self-conscious women do on beaches to avoid a boob popping out when putting on a bathing suit.)

During my couple of weeks as a guard, I spent most of my time counseling fortysomething men about other careers they might be qualified to do. One million men in the United States work as security guards.[18]

APPRAISAL TIME

"The grief in men has been increasing steadily since the start of the Industrial Revolution, and the grief has reached a depth now that cannot be ignored."[19]

Robert Bly wrote this in 1990. Since then, the economy has spun another rotation: we're in the midst of the high-tech revolution. How's that grief looking now?

Pretty sorrowful for the semiskilled and unskilled man. As factory jobs vanish, men lack the education—and perhaps aptitude—to make it in this new economy. In 1970s Britain, it used to be that 92 percent of working-age men (age sixteen to sixty-four) had a job; that's down to 76 percent.[20] In parts of the United States, like Madison Parish in the Mississippi Delta where the mill and farm jobs have disappeared, only 47 percent of prime working-age men are employed.[21] There is work at the two prisons and county jail in town—as guards.

Climb the socioeconomic scale to the lower-middle-class rung, where the small businessman, farmer, and artisan are battling to stop Walmart from eating them up and are highly vulnerable to the wider economic winds. In the "He-cession" of 2008–10, 80 percent of the jobs lost were men's.[22] Nearly a third of lower-middle-class families in the United States rely on food stamps or some form of benefits.[23] The middle-class man. Working his nuts off in that man-sapping office, using his education and nous to fit into this new way of working, but for what? Some have thrived, grown wealthy and powerful. But across the board, real income has fallen since the 1990s for the white middle-class man, and it's been flat since the early 1970s. "It literally takes two incomes, including the wife's, to earn what one income earned for a family forty years ago," Michael Kimmel notes in *Angry White Men*.

Put simply: "That 1971 family income was roughly the same as today's. . . . Then, it would have bought you a nice house in a good neighborhood with a decent school system, with about half left over for food and clothing and savings."[24] Just imagine prices staying the same but having your income doubled: that's the life the men before us had.

And those hitting the labor market now might come to marvel at the security we once had, where contracts were permanent and someone else chipped in for our pension. That infantilizing corporate structure—with people having a regular place to go to work—might even start to seem less absurd in retrospect. *Together we hold / On to our vision of global strategy / Oh KPMG.*

As for the top of the tree, there's no need to lose much sleep for these men. Some 95 percent of the Fortune 500 CEOs are male—as indeed are

98 percent of the self-made billionaires on the *Forbes* rich list.[25] It's like time froze during a golfing day for the Delta Kappa Epsilon class of 1971.

We've looked at lots of statistics, percentages, and macroeconomic patterns. But at the heart of each, there is a man who has to get up each morning and go to work—*if* he has a job—whose whole day will be heavily influenced by what he does for a living.

Whether he's bounding out of bed full of energy or perhaps lying there with a pit of anxiety in his stomach.

Whether, when he looks at himself in the shaving mirror, he likes what he sees—if it's someone who is living up to his expectations—or if he experiences a sinking feeling that the guy staring back isn't on track.

However long his commute will be, whether he has to live miles away from the nearest station just to find somewhere affordable or even whether he's in a city he wants to be in.

Whether he is spending his day doing the job he wants to do or just putting the hours in for the salary—when previous generations could have earned enough following a passion.

However those ten or so hours per day will be spent and who with. Whether he will laugh, sweat, feel any purpose and pride, or have to wade through resentment and frustrations. Whether he is likely to drink and smoke during the day.

Whether he'll return home to a partner or whether divorce has taken its toll; or whether he's the kind of blue-collar guy with no prospects whom women have decided they are just better off without.

If there are kids, whether he's able to spend enough time with them, be a laid-back dad, and meet their needs. Whether he's likely to have sex that night. The median frequency of sex has declined in the last twenty years from five to three times a month, with work presumed to be the main big factor.[26] And if he'll be able to get it up.

How well he will sleep that night.

That work has such a pervasive impact is borne out by the charity Mind, who has found the two biggest stresses in a man's life are directly related to what he does for a living: work and financial pressures. Both outstrip health and relationships worries, though, of course, work stress will affect these other two areas as well, for the mental clean sweep.[27] We've seen the terrible mental toll that work can take on men, depending on the other legs holding up his stool and how he's calibrated. Yet there are also extraordinary highs that can come from work: a real sense of power and purpose that can even trigger the libido to go into overdrive.

In the UK, men comprise 94 percent of the FTSE CEOs, yet also 95 percent of Britain's prison population.[28] Are we wired for this high–low crapshoot?

Dr. Helena Cronin, a rationalist philosopher from the London School of Economics, has been taking a good look at the Y chromosome:

> For males, they will tend to be overrepresented both at the top and the bottom of the heap. . . . Whether it's height or whether it's brilliance. This is something that Darwin noticed, and he noticed it not only for us but for all sexually reproducing species. But we don't really know exactly why.

Dr. Cronin has a theory:

> It seems to be something to do with competition. You can think of it this way. If you give a man fifty wives, he can have children galore. If you give a woman fifty husbands, it's no help whatsoever to her reproductive success. So over evolutionary time, men had to compete fiercely for mates. Women didn't.

131

Males, because they are fundamentally competing at everything all of the time with other males, put huge effort into being first and fastest, biggest and best—so when they fail, they just crash. That difference between males and females is so striking, I think of it as among males there are more Nobels but more dumbbells—and that is the story of males.[29]

RAGING BULLS

When all is going well, it is a similar feeling to sitting at the blackjack table with a nice pile of chips in front of you: competing and *winning*. It's energizing in the veins, you're just that little bit more gregarious at the table; you feel sexier and maybe even more generous. And so in life. The game feels good. And being a man, you attribute that success to how you've played your hand, not to luck.[30] It's your skill that's got you where you are; you deserve whatever status, money, power, or property you've accrued.

Conversely, when the chips are down, it replicates that slightly sickening, downbeat sensation of being on a losing streak with the cards. In life, men turn this frustration inward: they withdraw and isolate (more than women).[31] It's easier to shut down the emotional pores than be open to the stinging sensations of failure or the success of others. We get depressed, stressed, self-medicate, and self-destruct. When the hunter-gathering is coming up short, it's hard to feel like a man.

If failure—or thinking that we've failed—leads to an inward "crash," it also generates an outward energy: anger. An anger that is particularly acute now among white men, whose base level of expectation is an entitled sense that society and success is theirs for the taking. An anger that seems to blame others, often those who are perceived as being obstacles or rivals to their work success: immigrants, women, trade treaties, the purveyors of political correctness—and they're drawn to radical politics. Just as the downwardly mobile lower-middle class populated the Italian fascists and the *Kleinbürgertum* fueled the Nazis, so angry white males are driving Golden Dawn in Greece today and are among the Jobbik party members in Hungary calling for Jews to be put on a special register. An anger that is drawn to the regressively hypermacho: a Brazilian president who says of his five children: "There were four men; on the fifth I got weak and a woman came out."[32]

And, of course, closer to home, in Trump, a president who flaunts the red-meat masculinity and fuck-you freedom (reinforced by every more outlandish comment, tweet, or action that defies political gravity) that many men feel in such short supply of. For middle-aged men adrift in uncertainty, a blind tribal faith in a father figure who will magically conjure status and security back to the way they were—and keep (bogus) bogeymen at bay (if need be, with the promise of a physical barrier). A paternal figure, not even pretending to care for those outside the immediate clan, to mount on a modernity-defying pedestal. "I look at Donald Trump as like a model to me. I want to be like Donald Trump," a staunch supporter from Ohio told me.

That background hum of low-level rage crackles across radio call-in shows—72 percent of Rush Limbaugh's audience is male[33]—and simmers on the anti-women websites that are now listed in the Southern Poverty Law Center's annual hate survey.[34] And it's an anger that can erupt into terrible violence. "Going postal" is the explosive convergence of this man-work-anger nexus.

Between 1986 and 1997, more than forty people were murdered by current or former postal workers in at least twenty incidents. The macabre trend began at 7 a.m. on August 20, 1986, when Patrick Sherrill walked into the post office where he worked in Edmond, Oklahoma, and shot dead a supervisor who had disciplined him the night before. Within fifteen minutes, he'd killed fourteen coworkers before turning the gun on himself. The common thread that links this and the other murders that followed seems to be the cuts and efficiencies implemented by Reagan to streamline the US Postal Service. The workers who went on killing sprees were all post office workers who had been laid off, or downsized, or had their benefits slashed.[35]

Nor does "failure" have to wait until the workplace to morph into a murderous rage. Of the fatal school shootings carried out since 1987 in the US, all have been by boys—who have almost always been white.[36]

* * *

The workplace (and school) shootings seem to be the preserve of the white male. Kimmel terms these workplace shootings as "suicide-by-mass-murder"—a grandiose gesture that's rooted in an aggrieved entitlement, with a desire to make others pay.

"White men want to destroy the entire world in some cataclysmic video-game-and-action-movie-inspired apocalypse. If I'm going to die, then so is everybody else, they seem to say. Yes, of course, this is mental illness speaking: but it is mental illness speaking with a voice that has a race and a gender."[37]

He contrasts this with: "When young men of color experience that same sense of aggrieved entitlement—that perception of victimhood despite everything men expect for themselves—they may react violently, and even with lethal violence. But the victims of their violence are usually those whom the shooter believes have wronged him, and the unintended and accidental victims caught in the line of fire. And it rarely ends with his suicide."

By a beat-up main road in the north of Charlotte, North Carolina, away from the gleaming financial district that's second only to New York, Garry McFadden reflects on the twenty-two years he spent as a (black) homicide detective. "We're on what they call the Ford. Heavy African American populated area. We have a store over here called Mighty Midget Mart—that store has seen ten or fifteen homicides. Across the street, there were so many murders they changed the name of the street because it was that bad."

McFadden agrees with the notion that gang shootings tend to be a response to feeling slighted by someone in particular—rather than the grandiose gesture of aggrieved entitlement in a (white) mass shooting—or an attempt to prove manliness. "You gonna have to shoot somebody, you gonna have to make people scared of you, and to them that's being a man. But it's not."

The ex-cop now goes into schools to mentor at-risk boys. "All they want is somebody to care for them, to show them some love, give them some self-worth." And social mobility. Children born into the bottom fifth of household incomes in Charlotte have a mere 4.4 percent chance of reaching the top quintile at some point in their lives.

Chicago is perhaps a starker case in point. In a city where 92 percent of black sixteen- to nineteen-year-olds are unemployed, more than 80 percent of homicide victims were from the African American community in 2017.[38]

Nationally, the unemployment rate among blacks is about double that in the white community, as it has been for most of the past six decades.[39] For most, that will translate into the inward frustrations of being unemployed or a kick to self-esteem from doing a job that doesn't fulfill your potential.

If angry, white America is driven by desperate attempts to recoup the losses of what it once had, perhaps on the Ford the *loss* is of any pretense that the American Dream is an equal-opportunity employer. When a whole segment of society isn't able to "compete" on a level playing field in this great Y chromosome contest, this lack of employment opportunity fuses with a whole set of other complex issues—from biased policing to a dearth of male role models—to throw up destructive repercussions that ripple across society. Through schools, jails, mental health institutions, families, and neighborhoods. (In the UK, black men are also twice as likely to be unemployed as white males[40] and, lo and behold, have up to 60 percent higher depression rates.[41] They are three times more likely to be in jail.[42])

A week spent in court in Miami was to see twenty or so black guys shuffle in each morning, dressed in orange Dade County jumpsuits, chains rattling, to cursorily plead to a drugs charge before being shipped back to jail and into the spin-cycle of groundhog deprivation.

Guns. Sixty percent of gun owners in the United States are white males.[43] A testosterone patch clamped to the hips of fearful, angry men—to overcome the cravings for entitlement. Releasing a comforting fix of rugged freedom, no matter what shit job you're hostage to.

What began as whining about office life has somehow ended up in the intractable mires of US race relations and European fascism. But I guess that just serves to reinforce how critical work is to man, and, by extension, mankind. If one man's life can be so affected by what he does for a living—if it's *the* thing that is most likely to keep him up at night—then it follows that when that depth of feeling is aggregated across hundreds of thousands or millions of men, social movements can be unleashed. When more than half the young men in Spain are unemployed, alarm bells should be ringing. That black men in the US are as likely to be unemployed today as when Martin Luther King Jr. was alive, should be sounding the horn. More positively, the reduction in Catholic-male unemployment in Northern Ireland—especially the narrowing gap between that and Protestant unemployment—has been a core foundation in stopping peace from being blown off course.

Breaking the vicious cycle of male unemployment and generational violence: memo to the Middle East.

When those base male foraging instincts are suppressed, that gurgling masculinity pops out elsewhere. A thwarted desire to be productive can morph into the *de*structive. An inward self-destruction and an outward-facing anger. A susceptibility to whatever radical or toxic ideologies are in the ether. Why play by the rules of the competition when you can't even get a seat at the table? Why not hurl the table over?

BUSINESS PLAN

Finding a way to give a whole global swath of unemployed and underemployed men meaningful work and tackling the social disparities that have become so pronounced across the West, these are immense macroeconomic issues well beyond my pay grade and no doubt beyond the tangential reach of even the most well-intentioned global leader. But what those leaders—and bodies like the UN and EU—should urgently factor into their policy-making is that thwarted masculinity has serious social repercussions. When the economic opportunities aren't there, what else can make men feel like men?

Still beyond my station, I think, is how to at least make working life more tolerable for men. But if I were made Grand HR Poobah, those open-plan offices would cop it. Working spaces would be designed to foster productivity and creativity. A place to utterly concentrate (and meditate) but also that would allow passion to flow without being silently tutted at. When men were sent off for their personality makeovers from the 1920s, it was right that certain traits were discarded along with imperialism. There's no place for a bullying aggression; to be screamed at by a man or woman isn't much fun. But what's been filleted out from men are their maverick tendencies. I've seen so many *characters* across different sectors, often with brilliant ideas or genuine people skills, who have been spat out by corporate machines while the vanilla team player who doesn't rock the boat rises ever upward. Still more men self-censor their true characters—self-neutering with a shrug to climb the greasy pole and meet the mortgage payments.

My utopian HR department is also introducing Manual Labor Mondays. For those men who work in offices, every Monday morning they will put in a shift of physical work that benefits the community. Something to break that foraging physiology into a sweat and do something productive that has nothing to do with their career paths or identity. Get their RSI-inflicted hands dirty.

Men themselves need to take a look at the prevailing economic winds. If what's heading our way is more piecemeal work and fewer permanent contracts, a future where skills trump a strong pair of hands, how can we tether ourselves to avoid being blown away?

That may entail taking a deep breath and embracing jobs that traditionally are not seen as manly. Of the thirty occupations expected to grow fastest in the coming years, women dominate in twenty: the likes of nursing, medical secretarial work, and food preparation.[44] If we want to work in these growing sectors, some macho baggage might have to be shed.

Likewise, if maximizing family income is key, then it might have to be that men "sacrifice" their careers if the woman is the higher earner. And there's every chance she will be. In Britain, the number of higher-rate taxpayers (and those earning £1 million-plus) is growing faster among women than men,[45] while women are a third more likely to go to college than men. US campuses are already majority female and are heading in the same direction.[46] Not that any of this negates the current gender wage gap which, although narrowing and with multiple factors at play (including the likes of assertiveness), means US women earn around a fifth less than men.[47]

If a couples want to achieve their maximum possible income and have one of them at home to bring up the kids, then the day might be dawning when more and more men have to embrace being a stay-at-home dad.

Something I suspect won't come easily for quite a few: that's a lot of conditioning and hardwiring to overcome. Indeed, despite headlines suggesting that American men are swapping careers for childcare, "among two-parent households where women work, the percentage of men acting as the primary caregiver has actually *declined* slightly since the early 1990s."[48]

In this high-tech, high-uncertainty economy, men might also need to have an honest look inside their psyches to learn what's going to make themselves more robust. If, without those steady jobs for life, the work leg is going to always be wobbly, then how else can you make the stool secure? Maybe have more than one career option at the ready or know that something outside of work can also be a fulfilling source of status, identity, and community. Master a manly skill: another outlet to *do*.

And monitor what actually makes you happy, rather than what simply ticks the box of what you feel you *should* be doing. If you're a sensitive vervet-type prone to being affected by where you are in the surrounding pecking order, maybe be a bigger fish in a smaller pond. Question whether the urge to accrue as much money and cachet as possible is leading to genuine satisfaction, or whether it is driven by being a slave to the genetic impulse to maximize status and so enhance your reproductive odds.

As Yuval Harari says: "[People] choose what is good for the reproduction of their genes, even if it is bad for them as individuals. Most males spend their lives toiling, worrying, competing, and fighting, instead of enjoying peaceful bliss, because their DNA manipulates them for its own selfish aims."[49]

There are more ways than ever to keep your DNA happy. The economic climate might be more uncertain than our fathers experienced, but the times are also more flexible. It's an era in which you can reinvent yourself overnight, take your transferable skills and jump between jobs, and launch a business off a laptop. And if that hunter-gathering job spec is still running around your head, there'll be any number of reality TV shows more than happy to dump you on an uninhabited island.

WHAT SHALL WE WATCH TONIGHT?

When men were in crisis at the start of the twentieth century, popular culture threw up Tarzan and the cowboy legend. If there's any truth that "what we lose in reality we recreate in fantasy,"[50] then it's clear that those men, who'd been shepherded en masse into factories and offices, were pining for a return to primitive instincts or a rugged Western manliness. Indeed, the myth of the cowboy was invented *after* he had disappeared in reality. One of the fathers of this cowboy genre, Owen Wister, had actually been a broker who was sent to a dude ranch after having a brain-sprain breakdown.[51] The world he and others conjured up saw brave, skilled, stoic men conquering vast prairies that were free from feminization, workplace humiliation, and domestic emasculation.[52]

I spent a little time last year at cowboy college in Scottsdale, Arizona. Under the tutelage of Rocco, a New Yorker who was now every inch the bowlegged cowboy, I learned entry-level lassoing, cantering, and how to wrestle a calf. While I showed a surprising aptitude in handling a lasso, a wrestled calf came within an inch of landing a life-ending hoof on my soft city head.

As we sat around the ranch in the evening, the cowboys and me around a campfire, I ran through the basic should-I-have-life-envy checks. The sheer stunning beauty of the Arizonan landscape, the primordial pleasure of being around a fire and under the stars, the mastery of animal and environment, a raw masculinity that made me feel distinctly uselessly urban: all got ticks. That none of them had any women in their lives or could actually get their own thighs to touch: not great. But my abiding

envy was the freedom they reveled in. Rocco had no boss, no office politics, no appraisals or targets. He didn't care what anyone thought of him,
had no need to morph into a different version of himself, could provide
his own food, and had no physical boundaries between himself and the
open wilds. Maybe I should have stayed longer to de-sprain.

If men last century were fantasizing about escape, what reality are we
trying to re-create today? The fact that 135,000 people applied to be on
the latest series of *The Island with Bear Grylls* might alone speak volumes
about what our twenty-first-century heads are yearning for.[53] But what do
our viewing habits say about the inner male psyche? What are the male
archetypes we've created—the Tarzans and Buffalo Bills of today?

In crude terms, there are: the men who can operate by the escapist
codes of a different era or society (*Game of Thrones, Downton Abbey,
Rome*); men as part of a brotherhood (*Sons of Anarchy, Band of Brothers*);
and a very strong showing for maverick men who don't play by the rules
(*Breaking Bad, Narcos, The Wire, The Sopranos, Bourne*). None of which
are new genres—especially when allied to a good crime or power tale—
but perhaps show some of the enduring male fantasies. (*The Sopranos* was
also pioneering in speaking to the wider frailty of men.)

If there's one recent show, however, that captures the fantasy the modern male worker wants to recreate, I would posit that it's *Mad Men*. The
Wild West for our times is a 1960s Manhattan ad agency; Don Draper,
the John Wayne for today's open-plan office worker, vividly evoking an
era when men ruled the roost, sexual chemistry crackled, political correctness was a distant party-pooping nightmare yet to be invited, business
pushed at new frontiers, hedonistic behavior added to your own legend,
men looked like they were dressed for business, afternoons could be lost
to a bender, work stayed behind when you left the office, kids showed
deference and hats hadn't been hijacked by hipsters. And, above all, when
you had your very own office.

9
SET OUR
TESTOSTERONE FREE

FIGHT! FIGHT! FIGHT!

"It's not about hitting that guy. It's really about being hit. Can I take it? Can I feel it? Can I fucking feel anything in this world?"

Corporate finance guy in a dot-com

"You know, my whole life I'd never been in a fight. I never knew I could take a punch and get back up. I built my whole life around avoiding it, avoiding getting hit, avoiding confrontations, avoiding pain. . . . Once you know you can take a punch, you don't spend your whole life covering up."

A marketing guy in Silicon Valley[1]

There is *something* about fighting. Or even *nearly* fighting.

The one occasion in my life when I actually started a fight was more farce than *Fight Club*. Having been asked to give a talk at a synagogue at a Friday-night dinner—generally not a place of major pugilistic display—I duly spoke for forty-five minutes about some documentary highlights from my career. The first twenty minutes went well enough, but then I could detect murmurs, which grew into outright conversations breaking out at the tables. It was a losing battle as, being the Sabbath, there was no electricity—so no microphone and no hope of rising above the now full-scale chatter. I plowed on until the end and sat down to push the dairy-free trifle around my plate. It had been a long week. This wasn't the ideal way to unwind. Why couldn't they at least be polite enough to keep quiet when someone was giving up their time to do a talk they never even wanted to do? How can you make trifle without proper custard?

Some schmo then wanders over to my table and asks if he can have a word. *Sure.* We walk over to the buffet area. I brace for the usual request of whether I can get his daughter/friend some work experience.

I've done a lot of best man talks, he tells me. Which is nice for him.

The main thing is to keep them short.

Great. Thanks, pal.

And, you know, yours just went on too long. It was boring.

I was asked to speak for forty-five minutes—and that's what I did.

Yeah, you've really got to keep it shorter.

Right. So you feel the need to go up to someone who's given up his time, come here and given a speech, talked for as long as he was told to, to tell him his talk was too long and boring?

Well, I've done a best man speech and—

Are you a professional broadcaster?

No. But I've seen your work, and I think it's shit.

Maybe it was the rough week. The sheer insolence. The bruised ego from the chattering tables. The substandard dessert. But I just felt the red mist descend. Talking could no longer express what I wanted to convey.

My old school friend Dan was sitting on a nearby table. He said he had not seen a move like this since fifth form. He saw me reach over, yank the guy by his tie, and mouth the words, "Let's take this outside." As I pulled him by an ever-tightening knot toward the door, others dropped their pudding spoons to intervene. The great Friday night fistfight in a synagogue hall was averted. Schmo sat down, with profuse sweat patches breaking out under his pits.

But, I tell you, what a rush. What an affirming explosion of those fight-or-flight hormones actually being deployed not to leg it. My honor had been impugned, I'd been disrespected—and, for once, I acted like a brute man. I went home too pumped up to sleep. And awoke mightily relieved that we'd not progressed past tie pulling.

I get what drives the Silicon Valley guys to go to one of the real-life fight clubs that have sprung up in the wake of the film. After a day spent in a sanitized serotonin-sapping office, there's a need to feel *something*; to give those unreconstructed caveman hormones a run around the block. I felt this most not during my near handbags at dawn but in the ten days I happened to find myself on a Krav Maga course in northern Israel. With nothing better to do over a new year, my brother somehow talked two friends and me into going to learn this no-frills martial art, which was developed to fight off fascists in the 1940s and is now the de rigueur choice of inflicting maximum pain for not just the Israeli army but special forces around the world (and aped on screen by Bauer and Bourne). I should have sensed it wasn't going to be Club Med during the introductory session.

Hi, I'm Vlad. I work as a bodyguard in Moscow, and I'm here to learn new techniques for attack and defense.

I'm Vasily, I am mixed martial arts specialist and want to become harder for my job as bodyguard.

I am Dmitry [stares].

Hey, I'm Jake, I'm in the US naval reserves, and I've been doing karate for fifteen years and am a fifth Dan black belt.

Um, hi, I'm Tim. I've been doing yoga for about six years.

Ten days of getting punched, kicked, and strangled, being stabbed with fake knives and held up with fake guns, rebounding off the frames of the Russians, firing pistols, escaping carjackings, running down the beach while being barked at by ex-officers, and very occasionally landing the odd punch. A ten-day out-of-mind experience. I slept like a baby, made positive resolutions, found myself breaking out into the sort of spontaneous runs I'd only ever seen done by jocks on campus, and felt some intangible, undernourished roots of masculinity come back to life.

* * *

Man gets thrill from fighting: hardly the stuff of breaking news.

Any British market town on a Saturday night is a tinderbox of provincial menace where the wrong look can earn you a smack. At St. Andrews, such was the regularity that Etonians were punched outside the chip shop, I think the locals may actually have been following a roster. All part of an exemplary national tradition for mindless scrapping: in the early twentieth century, as many as half of working-class men might have been arrested for minor acts of violence or theft. As one bloke recalled, "When I was eighteen, I knew it took four things to be a man: fight, work, screw, and booze."[2]

France, naturally, applied more panache to its aggression. While turn-of-the-twentieth-century Brits were throwing haymakers in provincial pubs, Parisians were elegantly settling their disputes through duels, with as many as a dozen a week taking place in Paris.[3] Such was the prevailing code of honor that swords were drawn over the beauty of ladies' hands in Lille and the caliber of a horse in Strasburg.[4] Many duels were fought over women. When a Monsieur Charles de Bourg found his wife in bed with another man, he killed her, telling the court, "I was like a savage beast; when someone attacks my honor, I am the sort of man who is able to defend himself." The court acquitted him and chastised the other man for his cowardly behavior in not sticking around to defend the lady.[5] In 1967, while America got further sucked into Vietnam and the Middle East broke out into regional war, over in a French town a mayor and his rival deputy were squaring up for the country's last known duel.[6]

The aggression that's evident today tends to be somewhat less of the twenty-paces-at-dawn variety. That thwarted masculinity, as we have seen, can produce terrible work- and school-place shootings and cause gang-related homicides to spike in the US (bucking the wider trend across the West of falling violent crime).[7] At home, levels of domestic violence, although trending downward, appallingly still mean that one in four women experiences serious violence from an intimate partner during her lifetime.[8]

Incidentally, if there is a greater convergence between men and women—from a blurring of sexual behavior to increased numbers of women suffering from traditional male ailments like heart disease, perhaps due to work stress—then another of our less desirable traits may have rubbed off too. There are signs that female violence has increased, from rising assaults in Australia to violent crime carried out by women doubling in the last decade in the UK.[9] It's a violence that also pervades the home: males make up about 40 percent of the domestic abuse victims in Britain—some 800,000 men.[10] One in seven American men suffer serious violence from an intimate partner. Given the deep breath a bloke would have to take to walk into a police station to say his partner had been attacking him—and the terrible lack of male refuge places—who knows the true extent of men being abused by their wives or girlfriends? It's a crippling taboo that, just because it runs counter to our image of men, is barely on the radar.

Violence can leave a terrible trail in its wake, with families, neighborhoods, schools, and prisons left to pick up the pieces after men kick out against a lack of opportunity and an absence of ways to win esteem that don't entail a gun or gang. Despite women muscling in on assaults and wounding to narrow the gender gap, it's still mainly the preserve of men, who are arrested for around 80 percent of violent crime.

But let's park this nihilistic form of violence and return to the Silicon Valley guys staring at screens all day who feel alive again once blows are raining down on their heads; to the in-body oneness I experienced while trying to fend off simulated knife attacks from bestial bodyguards. Does this allude to a "good" aggression we should be indulging, something that's core to masculinity? Is man *supposed* to fight?

WIRED FOR WOOLLY MAMMOTHS

The Victorians certainly thought so, as they fretted about men becoming feminized and losing their imperial balls. So much so that they imbued male aggression with religious virtue, giving rise to the notion of Muscular Christianity. Jesus was recast by preachers as "the greatest scrapper who ever lived."[11] Manliness was next to godliness and an "antidote to the poison of effeminacy."[12] Organized sports were the cauldron in which to release this biblical bashing, where to be close to Jesus was to have your head stuck up against another bloody good chap's ass in the scrum. What began as British public schoolboys being sent to do noble battle on the rugby fields soon jumped to the United States and Australia and infused such movements as the YMCA and the Boy Scouts and contributed to the explosion of boxing, baseball, weightlifting, and athletics. One Frenchman was particularly moved after reading *Tom Brown's Schooldays*, a tale of boisterous bully-bashing, sport-obsessed life at an English boarding school, and visiting Rugby public school, which young Tom had fictionally attended and where the actual sport was invented: Baron Pierre de Coubertin, the founder of the modern Olympics.[13]

Those Victorians, whom I can thank for the enduring legacy of brutal cold showers at school, saw rough-and-tumble as key to bringing the best out of a man. For some, school games will invoke unremittingly bleak memories of preening jocks, fascistic PE teachers, and mouthfuls of mud. But what the Victorians tapped into is an enduring male yearning for risk and roughness. Nineteenth-century boys came up with a term for doing a dangerous deed for its own sake: doing "a stump."[14] Teenage boys in today's Northern Territories in Australia have a name for hammering cars off-road, often until they end up wrecks: "bush bashing."[15] That taxi drivers in Germany who had antilock brakes fitted then drove faster and crashed as much as before implies that there's a base level of risk we are drawn to (the theory of risk homeostasis, if you're wondering).[16] And it's a yearning that could stem from our wiring.

The University of Delaware psychology professor Dr. Marvin Zuckerman has found that there is a sensation-seeking genetic trait that drives people to take risks and, yes, it is more prevalent among men. Men score particularly highly on what he calls the thrill- and adventure-seeking traits.[17] To get scientific, the differences between a low and a high sensation seeker can be tangibly seen in diverging electrochemical reactions in the cortex of the brain and, biochemically, in levels of the monoamine oxidase enzyme. The risk-seeking tendency peaks in the late teens and early twenties and gradually declines with age, along with levels of testosterone.[18] This is not to say that all men are wired to be high-sensation seekers; there is a range, with most falling in the middle.

That we are drawn to drive fast, fight, or throw ourselves out of planes is rooted in the hunter-gatherer bodies we're still walking around in.

"In the past, sensation-seeking was found in just the struggle for survival," says Dr. Zuckerman.[19] "The hunting of large and dangerous game by men required a type of thrill- and adventure-seeking that also contributes to the success of the human race. Over the millennia, men also found in combat and war an outlet for their need for adventure.

"Mating, too, was a dangerous game that required risk-taking. The innate incest taboo drove men to seek mates outside their small groups, sometimes from unfriendly groups."

The woolly mammoths are gone, but we're still looking for that rush of blood. "Modern life, with its protected cultures and curtailment of war, has not wiped out the need for excitement. Some people find it through other people, in relationships and sex," he says. "Others need more of a thrill and go hang gliding or bungee jumping, although the most common everyday outlet for sensation-seeking is reckless driving. My work has shown that people have a basic need for excitement—and one way or another, they will fulfill it."[20]

While I tend to scooter around town at a sensible speed (other than when having infidelity dumped on me) and ski like a Floridian grandma, my older brother Mark is at his happiest when 23,000 feet up a mountain, riding his 1200 cc bike around a high-speed track, or free-falling out of a plane.

While our childhood upheavals turned me into an attention seeker, he became an archetypal sensation seeker. The daredevil edge has been blunted by having two kids and a full-on job, but, he says, "I've always loved things like high-altitude climbing. It's when I feel most alive and 'me.' I'm always a little depressed when I can't do them. It isn't an adrenaline addiction; on the contrary, I've always felt exceptionally calm when I'm hanging off an ice ledge or deep-water diving." (Indeed, it's that calm during moments of high sensation that makes these types good emergency workers.)

Today, more than ever, with our sedentary, sapping lifestyles, where can this "warrior energy"[21] find an outlet? How can that good aggression—and those risk-taking electrochemicals and enzymes—get a break in the modern world?

For boys, it might not be so easy. It's been a while since I read *Tom Brown's Schooldays*, but I don't recall any seven-year-old in it being suspended for throwing an "imaginary" grenade while making a *psshh* sound during playtime (as happened in Colorado)[22] or any other seven-year-old being suspended for chewing a Pop-Tart into the shape of a gun (Baltimore),[23] or a high school senior being expelled and questioned by police over common assault for custard-pieing a teacher on his last day of school (Altrincham, England).[24] Tom Brown may even struggle to get a game of rugger these days, given the 10,000 playing fields sold off in the eighties and nineties in Britain.[25] He'd be terribly disappointed with his chums in America, where only a quarter of children are getting enough exercise.[26] Don't get him started on obesity rates. And the opportunities to go rambling off on an adventure have been slashed: in a single generation since the 1970s, children's "radius of activity"—the area around their home where they are allowed to roam unsupervised—has declined by almost 90 percent.[27]

In a sign of the men they're destined to become, eleven- to fifteen-year-olds in Britain spend about half their waking lives in front of a screen.[28] Couch potato kid becomes sedentary office man or woman, who never breaks sweat during the day or feels on their back the sun that once baked the shirt of virtually all his ancestors. Long since disavowed of the once-heralded notion that business is the modern substitute for war: none of the bloodshed and devastation but all the same male virtues.[29] Too overworked, stressed, and unmotivated to get off the couch, let alone have sex. If ever two sets of figures were heading in the wrong direction during the last twenty years, it's these: while the average number of times a British man has sex each month has fallen from five to three, the number of American men who report doing no exercise at all has quadrupled (to 44 percent).[30] Four times as unfit, about half as likely to have sex. God bless progress.

In a southeast London boxing gym—stale sweat clinging to well-worn pads, newspaper cuttings of past triumphs yellowing on the walls—a former world champion is putting a bunch of men through their sparring paces. Duke McKenzie, still spry in his early fifties, bobs around the ring, holding up pads and issuing strangely soothing encouragement from behind his thick black-rimmed glasses. For most of us, managing to make a gym lesson is an achievement; for some of these guys, just being able to step out of the front door to come here is a serious triumph over crippling social anxiety. If ever there was an advertisement for the power of good aggression—to physically reconnect with our bodily design and hormones—it's here in Duke's gym.

Lee, six feet tall, tattooed, another bulky reminder that mental health problems defy any packaging, is one of the guys who have been referred to the gym by the charity Mind. The first three times he came here, he walked up to the door and then turned back. He is prone to serious depression and anxiety. "I can't leave the house. I will tend to lock myself away, even from my family. It's hard for me, and it's really hard for the family around me," says Lee of his darker days. "It can build up a lot of frustration about not being a real man—and not being able to do things for your family that others would consider normal."

After the fourth attempt, Lee hasn't looked back. Alongside the pills and talking therapy, the boxercise classes are now a staple of his treatment. "It helped me to realize that, yeah, I've got an illness, but I'm not really as worthless and useless as I thought I was. It has spurred me on—I'm starting to eat better, I'm sleeping better, my aggression where I might be snappy or blunt with people has subsided.

"The biggest thing is that I've actually started to like myself again— 'cause I can see that I'm achieving something. This sort of thing should be given on prescription."

Duke, who has KO-ed twenty opponents on the way to world titles at three different weights, sees a lot of men and boys from all backgrounds pass through the gym. And he sees a lot of anger.

"I've got a lot of angry men in my gym, there's no doubt about it. Life makes people angry. It puts pressure on men they can't deal with. There's a lot of people who can't pay bills, and many with people or family issues," he says. "Here, they can take out their angst, whatever natural aggression they've got in their system, in a positive way."

WAR AND THE PIECES

Our muscular Victorians would have approved of Duke's gym.

At the end of the "Fight" chapter in *Tom Brown's Schooldays*, the author, Thomas Hughes—himself a boxing coach—urges boys to avoid fights, "But don't say 'No' because you fear a licking, and say or think it's because you fear God, for that's neither Christian nor honest. And if you do fight, fight it out; and don't give in while you can stand and see."[31]

Others saw mere fighting as not enough; true male values could only be forged in war. Future President Theodore Roosevelt, having faced down his neurasthenia at a dude ranch in the Dakota Territory, wrote in 1895, "This country needs a war."[32] He argued: "The greatest danger that a long period of peace offers to a nation is that of [creating] effeminate tendencies in young men."[33] The 65 million men who, not long after, would fight in the First World War—and the nine or so million who never returned—could consider themselves suitably defeminized.

One of those millions, cocooned in a desperate trench by No Man's Land, wrote: "Amid these surroundings, aided by wet and cold, and every minor discomfort, I have found happiness and content such as I have not known for many months."[34] That was Winston Churchill. Having been humiliated by the failure of his Gallipoli campaign, Churchill quit his post as first lord of the admiralty, plunged into one of his deep depressions, declared himself finished—and then asked to be sent to the front line. It was there, in this crucible of human horror, that Churchill came back to life.

"I think a curse should rest on me—because I love this war. I know it's smashing and shattering the lives of thousands every moment, and yet, I can't help it, I enjoy every second of it," he wrote to a friend in 1916.[35]

Churchill is far from being alone in finding exhilaration amid the grisliest conflicts. The screenwriter William Broyles Jr. served with distinction in Vietnam. Despite the brutality and futility, he wrote later, "I miss it because I loved it, loved it in strange and troubling ways." He tried to break down "why thoughtful, loving men can love war even while knowing and hating it." Among the reasons why, he deduced:

- Part of the love of war stems from its being an experience of great intensity; its lure is the fundamental human passion to witness, to see things, what the Bible calls the lust of the eye and the Marines in Vietnam called eye fucking. War stops time, intensifies experience to the point of a terrible ecstasy.
- War replaces the difficult gray areas of daily life with an eerie, serene clarity. In war, you usually know who is your enemy and who is your friend, and are given means of dealing with both.
- War is a brutal, deadly game, but a game, the best there is. And men love games. You can come back from war broken in mind or body or not come back at all. But if you come back whole, you bring with you the knowledge that you have explored regions of your soul that in most men will always remain uncharted. Nothing I had ever studied was as complex or as creative as the small-unit tactics of Vietnam. No sport I had ever played brought me to such deep awareness of my physical and emotional limits.[36]

When Teddy Roosevelt declared that the United States "needs a war," his was the generation that venerated those who had fought in the Civil War thirty years before. When a young college-bound writer, Phil Caputo, volunteered for Vietnam, he was visualizing the derring-do of the men who'd fought in the Second World War twenty years earlier: "I saw myself charging up some distant beachhead, like John Wayne in *Sands of Iwo Jima*, and then coming home a suntanned warrior with medals on my chest."[37] We are all weaned on the idea that fighting for your country—being willing to sacrifice your life for the greater good—is the ultimate act. And the apex of masculinity. "Gee, I wish I were a man. I'd join the Navy,"[38] a First World War recruiting poster put it bluntly; today, the British army exhorts young men to "Be the Best," while the US Army is searching for a new slogan as effective as the 1990s' "Be All That You Can Be." Men before us faced down fascism; how can we possibly do anything as meaningful or heroic?

Which perhaps explains why we can't seem to let the Second World War leave our imaginations. This decade already, more than fifty World War II movies have been released, bringing the total out there to more than 1,300 (far outstripping any other conflict and ten times the number of First World War films).[39] For all the major conflicts that have followed—Korea, Suez, Vietnam, Afghanistan, Iraq—the 1939–45 war remains the last pure expression of good versus evil, man fending off an existential threat to our homes and countries. Tellingly, in the decade when we went into Iraq and got bogged down in Afghanistan, the number of World War II films more than doubled: from eighty-six in the 1990s to 180 in the 2000s. An anchor of certainty amid the military and moral chaos. And perhaps keeping the flame of *war = heroism* cinematically burning helps induce enough young men to sign up for the dwindling number of posts the military needs to fill these days.

"We have the disadvantage that we actually have no wars on," said the boss of the company hired to recruit soldiers to the British Army, when pushed to explain to politicians why recruitment numbers were seriously down. "Soldiers like to join the army when they actually have something to do. . . . You can pull faces at me but actually it is something that is factually true."[40] Were his equivalent in ISIS being grilled before their version of the genteel parliamentary select committee, I suspect no one would be pulling miffed faces at him. An estimated 40,000 foreign recruits, including around 300 from the United States, traveled to Iraq and Syria to swell the ranks of the local ISIS fighters.[41] In the United States, the army reported falling 6,500 troops short of its recruiting target for 2018.[42]

It's impossible to say what motivated a young man—the typical foreign jihadi was a male between eighteen and twenty-nine[43]—to leave Belgium, Germany, Denmark, France, Britain, or America and head to Kobani, Syria, to set up a caliphate. There is no single "pathway" to becoming a terrorist; no socioeconomic background, no level of religious upbringing—though the zeal of the convert is seen as a factor.[44] I would imagine that some sort of repressed, or twisted, masculinity should be thrown into the mix. Alienated young men, maybe with repressed sex lives, yearning for respect or significance, who have drunk in the militaristic heroism portrayed in shared online clips—films that hit the same warrior trigger that the *Sands of Iwo Jima* once activated for our Vietnam vet.

An airport security photo of five young men from Portsmouth—the "Pompey Lads"—snapped at Gatwick, looks like any group of Top Man or Gap guys on their way to a guys' holiday or stag. They flew to a Turkish resort and then slipped into Syria to join the fight. Of the five, four died—including a supervisor at a national clothing chain—and the other was jailed in Britain after cutting short his jihad on day seventeen (having been put on underwear-washing duties).[45] The jockstrap washer revealed that he'd wanted to call their group the Britani Brigade Bangladeshi Bad Boys. It would almost have been comic had the Bad Boys not been on their way to join the most barbaric, demonic group seen since the Nazis.

If proving their manhood was their thing, ISIS has pushed hypermasculinity into savage overdrive: systematically raping and committing sexual violence against captured girls and women, trafficking women to work in de facto brothels, issuing guidelines that it is "permissible to have intercourse with the female slave who hasn't reached puberty if she is fit for intercourse," throwing gay men off buildings, humiliating Western male captives, and even setting up marriage centers where women can sign up to wed a fighter.[46]

One doesn't want to come up with too many factors and explanations for why someone becomes a terrorist; not only is it guesswork, but it can also almost feel like it takes free will out of the equation: that they are "products" of situations rather than men who have willingly decided to get on a plane to wage jihad. But, if we are trying to explain the allure of ISIS, I sense that broken or bastardized masculinity has to be factored in.

If those young men breezing through the south terminal of Gatwick in their shades and casual clothes thought that they were off to fight for an ideological cause—their version of the International Brigades who went to Spain to take on the nationalists in the 1930s—then it is interesting to see scores (maybe even hundreds) of other Westerners heading to the same war, with the same rationale, but joining the other side. City traders, teachers, a surf instructor from Florida, and many former soldiers—who openly admit to missing combat—who went to fight alongside Kurdish forces against the Islamic State. A photo of a foreign legion of anti-ISIS fighters shows a dozen or so maverick-looking guys lined up for a football squad–style snapshot, in various states of uniform, proudly holding rifles aloft. It already has a sepia World War II feel to it.

Fighting ISIS: it's the closest a man can come today to battling against unambiguous evil. To do what so many generations of men have done before: put your life on the line for a greater cause. To give those risk-taking tendencies an honorable outlet. (Which is all now being reflected on screen in a profusion of shows about the SEALs and other special units, joining the traditional World War II fare of good vs. evil.)

"I was sitting at my desk in London, in an ordinary job, working in the City. Every day I'd flick on my computer screen and see the most horrendous crimes being committed in the Middle East. It just stirred me into action."[47]

Harry, a former private boarding schoolboy, gave up his desk job as a trader, and, with no previous military training, flew to join the Kurdish People's Defense Unit. He kept a grenade in his pocket, in case ISIS was about to take him captive.[48]

"I was ready to die and kill. I knew what I was getting myself into. I spent five months there. I saw a great deal of fighting and took part in two large operations. Islamic State shot at me, I shot at them.

"The people we were up against in the Islamic State, well, they are barbaric. People will understand why I went out."[49]

STILL BATTLING

At a serene country house off the M25 in Surrey, twenty miles south of London, a group of men sitting around in a circle are struggling to understand why *they* went out. Why they went out to Iraq, Afghanistan, Bosnia, Belfast, the Falklands, and what they came back as.

If ever you feel a macho flicker that war might be romantic, spend a few days at the charity Combat Stress. If ever a president or prime minister wants to see the human cost of sending troops into battle, sit in on a therapy session run by the charity.

Hear a sailor who was aboard the HMS *Sheffield* when it was sunk more than thirty years ago during the Falklands conflict describe how, on some days, it's still "complete carnage inside my head. . . . My war isn't over." Listen as Frank, who spent eight years as a paratrooper in Northern Ireland, relays how recently he dived to the floor in a café thinking he'd seen a sniper, when in fact it had been someone opening a window opposite. Sit with Alex, a former Royal Engineer who served in the first Gulf War, Rwanda, and the Balkans, as he tells you that sometimes his head hurts so much he just has to sit down and sleep.

Or spend just a little time at VA hospital in Chicago watching a Vietnam vet paint a paper mask to try and express—and purge—the emotions that still torment him decades later. Or wander over to the National Veterans Art Museum in the city to see the terrible scars of conflict brought to hauntingly beautiful life in works of art and sculpture.

Men whose days and nights are still utterly affected by the battles, carrying the psychological wounds of PTSD, with its flashbacks, anxiety, depression, and the accompanying drug and alcohol abuse used to dull the pain. An epidemic that afflicts veterans across the United States.

Since 9/11, some 2.77 million service members have been deployed.[50] The Department of Veterans Affairs estimates that 11–20 percent of those who served in Iraq and Afghanistan suffer from PTSD in a given year.[51] That equates to somewhere between three hundred thousand and half a million or so vets with PTSD, and that's before you factor in Desert Storm, Korea, or the quarter-million Vietnam vets who are *still* traumatized.[52]

Behind each statistic is a hero in enduring pain. At Combat Stress, Frank told me he went through thirty self-abusive years before he sought help and his PTSD was diagnosed. Many ex-soldiers were never able to ask for or receive help. More Falklands veterans have taken their own lives since the war than actually died in conflict. That's already the case for the American, British, and Australian forces who fought in Afghanistan.[53] Indeed, such is the immediacy of the psychological strain of these distant wars with their ambivalent rationale and support back home that in 2012, the number of *active duty* US soldiers who killed themselves, 177, exceeded the 176 who were killed while in the war zone.[54] The trauma of war was deadlier than the Taliban. Surely, it's a national scandal that every day in the United States, some twenty veterans will take their own lives.[55]

At VA hospitals and groups like Combat Stress, alongside the traditional talking and pill therapies, another approach is being used to help heal the psychological scars: art. Any residual macho stereotypes are left at the door of the art room, where classical music plays gently in the background, as a group of vets in rapt concentration are sketching abstract charcoal images and pencil drawings of whatever festering image of war has percolated to the surface, using art to dislodge that entrenched trauma, which can then be talked through. Some of the artwork hanging on the walls is beautifully haunting. Alex, the Royal Engineer, has produced mesmerizing sculptures expressing the feeling of being trapped.

Steve, a light infantryman whose PTSD went undiagnosed for seventeen years, has painted a lurid, snarling skull. "When I'm painting, the thoughts and flashbacks don't come in. There's been points in the last three years when I just wanted to do away with myself—and without the art and the support, I just wouldn't be here."[56]

Caesar's view that war is inevitable—a result of man's inherent aggressiveness—prevailed for centuries. Across Europe and the New World, battle was seen as the universal rite of passage for entering manhood; on the eve of the First World War, conflict was still being talked about as a biological necessity.[57]

If we do have some sort of biological urge to wage war—rooted in our hunter-gathering, sensation-seeking DNA—then our conquering of that instinct is a mark of civilization. No longer drawing your sword when a Frenchman insults your horse is a sign of progress, I'd say. That levels of violence have fallen across the West, for a complex set of reasons—maybe even including removing lead from gasoline[58]—can only be a good thing. Merely walking through the door of Combat Stress is to be thankful that countries at least give mediation a go at the UN before dashing balls first into battle.

Nor can we assume that it was just our genes all along prodding us into battle. There are times when it is in a country's interests to whip up a macho frenzy. France pushed the whole honor and ritual combat shtick as a reaction to being defeated by Germany—and worrying about Germany's superior resources and population: manly courage became a national resource to urgently cultivate.[59] British schoolboys were similarly being urged to embrace the noble virtues of being concussed in a rugby scrum at a time when the Indians were starting to rebel and the Zulus had given Her Majesty's forces a bloody routing. The military threats a country faces—or whatever imperial ambitions it might harbor—will affect just how far macho values are prized in a society. The United States still likes its leaders to look good in a pair of cowboy jeans; Russia opts for more of the khaki trousers and topless-on-horseback look. Switzerland has seemingly made as many films about Heidi, the Alpine orphan girl, as war.[60]

Just as with our sexual instincts, we might not be slaves to how we are wired, but let's not discount the fact that releasing aggression, taking risks, seeking out-of-the-ordinary sensations, battling for a greater good, and even fighting on the front line will make some of us feel that we're living. Make us feel like men, not mechanized cogs on a factory floor or aimless apes trapped in offices. "I was excited by the idea that I would be sailing off to dangerous and exotic places after college instead of riding the 7:45 to some office," recalls one Vietnam vet.[61] A yearning so deep that Alex, the ex–Royal Engineer, says he'd go back to the army in a shot, despite the night sweats and noise in his head.

Recognizing that men—especially before testosterone starts to flag—can have this inner drive means we can at least think about ways to indulge it without resorting to crashing a car, committing violent crime, joining a gang, or signing up for the army on a false promise. We can factor in that it's a potent force that can be harnessed to get those three core brain chemicals firing, with positive aggression able to help soothe mental woes or boost self-esteem when the economic means aren't there.

So what to do with this knowledge?

FIGHT THE POWER

As individuals, maybe positive aggression should be a core leg of the stool keeping us steady. Perhaps working up a serious sweat and expressing a controlled form of risk aren't just nice also-haves to the workweek but should be fundamental chemical connections. Prescribe punching therapy with Prozac.

For our boys and young men, there's a compelling need to elevate the physical beyond the hour or two a week they get if they're lucky. Schools could be flooded with more sports and martial arts. Not just the usual ball-centric stuff but any discipline—team, individual, or even yoga—that a boy or young man can connect with. The impact on even the most wayward kids, often already with a criminal record or history of absenteeism, is striking. A study in Chicago found that when these at-risk kids committed to a program of after-school sports—like wrestling, archery, or boxing—coupled with one hour a week of group counseling, there was a 44 percent reduction in violent crime. The program cost $1,100 per participant but saved the community an estimated $3,600 to $34,000 per person in crime-related costs.[62]

If a national sports and martial arts program for schools were also extended to take in men (and women) without work—who could be incentivized to attend through bonus payments/vouchers—then surely this would pay for itself in reduced unemployment benefits, obesity, and mental health treatment and criminality costs. Not to mention the feel-good factor that would be generated.

If, given the levels of youth unemployment and obesity and the insecure job market that awaits, we're really going for the full nanny-state screw-austerity intervention, maybe it's time to look to those who know a thing or two about keeping aggressive tendencies under wraps: the Germans. For years, Germany offered young men *Zivildienst*, civilian service, as an alternative to the mandatory military national service (both were scrapped in 2011). At its peak, 130,000 young people were posted to work in retirement homes, hospitals, and facilities for disabled people for a year.[63] Wiping the asses of German grannies might be a tough sell compared to a day on the Xbox. Yet if some sort of national service could be devised that had nothing to do with the military but was instead rooted in physical fitness, being part of some wider group with an identity and mentors, learning a skill, and doing communal good at the same time, then maybe it's worth a shot.

MEN ON A MISSION

Which I think alludes to something more fundamental. Fighting doesn't have to be literal. There is intense meaning and belonging that can come from fighting for a cause. Tapping into the tribal instincts of battling for something bigger than yourself: from the sense of "brotherhood" that used to prevail in the mutton-chopped days of 40 percent union membership to the electrifying current thrown up by the Arab Spring, to the youthful passion of the #NeverAgain movement spurred by the awful high school shooting in Parkland, Florida. Men and women on a mission—and brought to life.

There is something intoxicatingly meaningful about fighting for something you believe in. And you're willing to take more risks in pursuit of that cause. Despite being a hypochondriac who always travels with two paracetamol in my pocket, I've ended up in some fairly hairy situations in the line of campaigning journalism. To expose anti-Muslim sentiment in Northern Ireland, I worked undercover in a Belfast kebab shop in a Real IRA area, pretending to be one of the Afghan workers who'd been receiving abuse for months. Having not learned the finer art of kebab carving, all I could do was push a broom around and do my best to look like I'd just come from Kabul. One night a group of guys came in and started hurling abuse at me. *Go back to Bam Bam land . . . Paki sheep.* Eventually one leaned over the counter and spat directly in my face. Horrific to have someone's gob in your face, awful to know this was the sort of thing the Muslims had been putting up with for months, yet strangely satisfying to see that my hidden camera had caught the arc of the spit beautifully and those young men would soon be headlining BBC news.

At least when I went across the Caribbean to try to track down clues for who the real murderers were in the case of Kris Maharaj—the innocent British guy who has been in jail in Miami since 1986, with the incredibly supportive wife—I tended to have a bodyguard with me. Whom I was more than grateful for when, after being busted secretly filming a drug dealer in the Bahamas, we found the car battery had gone dead. If you think that you can make a difference to an innocent man who faces dying in prison, then some risks are worth taking. Such is the passion of Kris's lawyer, Clive Stafford Smith, that I've seen him head off deep into Colombian cartel territory in search of that killer piece of evidence to set Kris free.

This isn't some preachy call for everyone to be out there fighting—coming from someone who has had the chance to be part of a culture at the BBC where people are committed to making a difference (especially a certain shouty boss woman) and some really do put their necks on the line to expose what's going on in the world. When we were being urged to *start a revolution,* we had twice the real income, bags more spare time, and were part of big movements, like unions, with whom we could tag along. Yet the inequality today is back to where it was when "Revolution" was recorded in 1968.[64] Nowadays, though, it's hard enough to do anything other than fight to keep a job, hang on to the property ladder, and get the kids into a half-decent school. But as we go through life looking to keep those three brain chemicals nicely abundant, find some sort of meaning beyond our own comfort and ego, and throw a few bones to the inner male desire to fight, then there's a lot to be said—whether through work or outside—for summoning the inner Lennon.

If I were to bite the dust next week, as my life flashes before me—the terrible dates, the wasted health-care payments—I think the experience I'd derive most pleasure from would be the fight to give lonely old people a voice. How we treat the elderly is a disgrace. They are parked in front of the TV in stinking, claustrophobic old people's homes; trapped in high-rise flats not seeing anyone for weeks at a time; and beset by loneliness, malnourishment, and rampant untreated depression. I wanted to show that these older people, beyond the wrinkled packaging, are just the same as you or me: individual characters with passion and humor who can't believe the age they've reached. As we filmed in nursing homes and bingo halls, the idea struck to do something that would challenge our preconceptions of the elderly and also take them on a life-affirming rock-and-roll journey: form the world's oldest rock group. We brought together forty or so of the lonely old people out of their apartments and residential care homes to the old Beatles studio at Abbey Road to do a cover version of, what else, "My Generation." Our lead singer, Alf, a ninety-year-old with two remaining teeth who'd always dreamed of being a theatrical star, belted out "I hope I die before I get old." Thus were born The Zimmers, with a combined age of more than three thousand years.[65]

They became an overnight global sensation, going to number one on YouTube. Alf and the band rocked around the world—to the fifty-plus countries that covered their story, to legions of screaming fans in Germany, to primetime America alongside George Clooney on *The Tonight Show with Jay Leno,* even to the UN. I saw a ninety-year-old man's dreams come true, even though that meant he had to jump out of a wheelchair to strut around onstage as a beige-clad Roger Daltry before collapsing back into the chair. Alf knew this was no dress rehearsal. Beyond the razzmatazz—not least seeing Winnie, 99, door-stepped outside the BBC by two South Korean TV crews—the true pleasure came from the lasting bonds and loneliness-busting friendships that formed among the band. When Alf passed away at ninety-three, his coffin disappeared behind the curtain to the sound of his version of "My Generation" blasting through the crematorium, fellow band members shuffling to the music in the pews. Even the vicar boogied.

Shortly before he died, Alf told me that he could now die a happy man. No amount of tie pulling can match that.

QUALITY MAN TIME

"It is, unlike marriage, a bond that cannot be broken by a word, by boredom or divorce, or by anything other than death."[66]

Phil Caputo wrote this ten years after coming home from Vietnam a shattered man—not the suntanned John Wayne figure he'd envisioned when enlisting. The bond he talks about is the camaraderie felt among the men in his infantry battalion; a "tenderness" that led two of his friends to die while trying to save the corpses of men from the battlefield. It is common to hear from soldiers that when they're actually fighting, it's not about patriotism or some lofty ideal but the love and loyalty they have for each other. What fellow Vietnam vet William Broyles Jr. described as "a love that needs no reasons, that transcends race and personality and education—all those things that would make a difference in peace. It is, simply, brotherly love."[67] The brothers in arms might even be releasing the same hormone, oxytocin, that makes new mothers feel protective.[68]

But away from the intense life-and-death crucible of war, is there something distinct and vital about male friendship—a peacetime facsimile of that camaraderie? And do we get enough man time these days to express it?

Pissing on fires together to douse the flames as the cavewomen looked on in awe at our mastery of nature may have been the root of male bonding for Freud.[69] Firefighting aside, we need each other: man is far too funy to kill big beasts on his own. It's fine to be an antisocial orangutan when you're happy to eat mainly fruit, spiced up with the odd termite or piece of bark. If you want antelope, gazelle, or wildebeest steak, though, then we have to cooperate with each other.

From the Stone Age to the Bronze Age to the Iron Age and beyond, man has spent most of his time with other men. School, work, and social lives have predominantly involved males around males. And when women began to encroach into our lives—in the workforce, at church, making homes more female—men's reactions were to create women-free spaces: pubs, saloons, fraternities, and sports teams flourished. In England, there was one pub per one hundred people in the eighteenth century (ten times the number now).[70] One in four American men belonged to a fraternity lodge in 1900[71]—comfy places that re-created the very feel of home, bar the presence of a woman.[72] When women did breach the male bastion of the pub, there was clear gender delineation well into the 1970s.

"Women in pubs were accepted initially when they were there with their men. Friday night was when you went out with the boys, Saturday night with the missus—and there were rules about it. . . . And the female drinker was expected to stay in her designated area."[73]

The Grill bar in Aberdeen only allowed in women as of 1976, when compelled by the Sex Discrimination Act—but didn't install a women's toilet until 1998.[74]

Half the married men I know have to get a "pass" to get a night out. The idea of every Friday being a night with the boys would be too laughable to even raise with other halves while trying to keep a straight face. The pub itself is an endangered species: the rowdy boozer swept aside by the relentless gastromarch, with menus "typed" in Courier and artisan relish masquerading as ketchup. Twenty-one thousand British pubs have bitten the sawdust since 1980.[75] Its sticky-floored trans-Atlantic cousin, the bar, also appears to be heading toward the endangered watch list—with the *Boston Globe* lamenting the loss of twenty of the city's finest bars in a mere five years.[76]

If the pub, bar, or craft microbrewery is now the domain of the hand-cut beer-battered French fry, that other reliable stronghold of masculinity, the soccer/football field, is playing home to the "prawn sandwich brigade" (to invoke former Manchester United midfielder Roy Keane's bile for the corporate hospitality nonfans—"shrimp sandwich" to you Americans). Soccer fields in the UK used to be a sensory assault: being tossed around the bobbing terrace, deafened by a chant boozily delivered down your ear, scalded by gloopy beef drinks, someone's smoke wafting back into your face, and, when Leeds were in town, someone's two-pence coins landing on your head. It was where I first tasted the exotic aroma of cigar smoke and swearing as a kid; where the smell of horse manure became synonymous with a heightened sense of danger. When I go to a soccer field today, I feel like I'm a spectator rather than being part of the beast as I once was.

When fans at a number of clubs were recently caught singing "Get your tits out for the lads," it was such a daft, retro form of tabloid sexism it struck me as blokes clumsily kicking back at the sanitized stadium they were sitting in. A stadium in which they could once stand, drink, smoke, project menace—and actually afford to go to every game if they were working-class. "Get your tits out," the oafish warbling cry of an endangered species.

Woe is man. He can't go to the pub or bar anymore, can't throw a dart without hitting a kale fry, can't escape the missus without her permission, can't stand on the piss-reeking bleachers singing vulgar songs. Even golf is in decline, as divorced dads forgo their eighteen holes on a Saturday to see the kids.[77] Before this turns into an episode of *Bring Back the Seventies* or *I Miss Misogyny*, let's state the obvious: some of this represents real progress. Men spending more time with their families, more egalitarian marriages, sports becoming less sexist, bars that serve edible food, and deaths during fraternity hazing no longer being seen as par for the Sigma Alpha Epsilon course.

So why the semisad face?

Well, some of the rough-and-tumble is good for us. Bars, sports events, etc., have been places where, to quote those fifteenth-century Feast of Fools theologians, the barrels of wine can let in air so they don't explode. Considering how crazy men go on stag/bachelor weekends (no longer just nights out) these days, you can see that's a lot of built-up air. The traditional male crucibles were places where some of that pent-up aggression and testosterone could be regularly released in bursts (especially important now that work, for most, offers scant opportunity for this). When not released, that stale air can start to take on a bad smell—as sociologist Michael Kimmel found in a Brooklyn bar that had been home to generations of firefighters that he quotes: "Those bitches have taken over. They're everywhere. . . . There's nowhere you can go any more—factories, beer joints, military, even the goddamned firehouse! [Raucous agreement all around.] We working guys are just fucked!"[78]

Should our ranty fireman have been looking for some empirical justification for being fucked, he could have called on a study carried out in Scotland. The research—as far as I know, not commissioned by a particular pub in Aberdeen—found that going to the pub with friends was beneficial to men's mental health (though not necessarily so great on the physical side).[79] What the *bona fide* Glasgow Caledonian University study concluded was that the pub was crucial for how middle-aged men formed and sustained friendships—"If you don't go to the pub, you'd never see anyone"—buying a round was an essential part of the ritual ("the male equivalent of a friendship bracelet"), and the alcohol allowed men to open up and express emotions. Not the traditional national pastime of Scottish men.

Callum: Men don't really like to open up or chat as easily, so they
need a couple of pints to try and kind of get them oiled

168

up. . . . Women I think are more naturally kind of gregarious and bubbly and sociable, so they don't really need to be drunk.

Hugh: Drinking with these guys over the years has probably saved my mental health on numerous occasions.

Callum: If you go out with your mates, have a few drinks, it's great for your mental health. You don't feel lonely, you don't feel sad or depressed, it always cheers you up, you know.[80]

So perhaps we should see quality man time as another vital leg of the stool. There's a serious therapeutic underpinning to making sure men carve out enough time to spend with each other. As the relationship gurus have stressed, as well as giving our partners space, we need to be kind and generous to their needs—and that need might well include some regular time with male friends. And of course women might need time with their girlfriends. (Look, how much more of a case do I have to build to get you guys more passes?)

By the way, the real revelation from the study came when one Glaswegian admitted in front of his mates that he drank *rosé wine*, but only behind closed doors: "And I could handle it, I mean, behind closed doors in the company of close friends, but not if I'm out in the pub, no."

I have some extraordinary female friends. Women I confide in, laugh with, learn from—and utterly love being around. I couldn't live without them. But there is something different you get from being with a group of close male friends. There's a different energy and humor. Life feels lighter when you're with them. Problems that have been building in your head can be lanced with a well-aimed, often brutal joke that realigns perspective. Maybe it's a tribal thing: feeling safer and bolder with a protective pack around. Maybe it taps into the way we've been living since we decided a fruit and bark diet wasn't going to cut it. Perhaps it's just being able to release the innate immaturity that was instilled at an all-boys' school. But when I get to hang out—alas, not that often given the mass suburban exodus—with my closest male friends as a group, I feel centered; the world makes more sense.

To lapse into the candor of a Glaswegian drunk on rosé, you can feel something akin to that battalion "brotherly love" for friends. Friends whose problems become yours, who'd you take a bullet—well, a punch—for, and where it transcends that traditional sense of competition that shimmers beneath the surface of many a male friendship (we might have agreed to cooperate on snagging a wildebeest, but it was still head-to-head on the mating front). Morrissey might have sung that we hate it when our friends become successful. But not always, I'd say.

10
SPARE PART ON A PORN SET

WHY MEN REALLY NEED TO GET A GRIP

On Venice Beach, nonagenarian Alf and I did have a little chat about fake breasts, a phenomenon he'd somehow failed to come across between the bingo hall and bus to the supermarket. But for all his carpe diem and genteel open-mindedness, I suspect he might have been a little overwhelmed if he'd accompanied me on one of my next trips back to Los Angeles.

The four phases of being on a porn set.

One: awkwardness. Feeling like you shouldn't really be there while a young dark-haired woman in a green bikini is in prescene discussion with the director.

Actress: Just nothing in my butt.
Director: Nothing in your butt. What about slapping, choking?
Like that, or you don't?
Actress: That's fine.
Director: You, you like it? If you like it, tell me, we'll do it in a scene. Slap me or choke me, and he'll do it, otherwise he won't do it. You ready?

Two: titillation. The inner teenage boy cannot quite believe he's a few feet away from the actress having baby oil poured over her ass by a Frenchman who swiftly dispenses with the bikini and gets to work—taking her through the basic continental buffet of porn positions (he pulls Gallic puppy dog eyes to ask if he can *"eat ze ass"* but is politely rebuffed).

Three: boredom. After half an hour, all eroticism has drained from the room. It's like watching a hackneyed pantomime at a regional theater: *he's* (doing you from) *behind you*. I find that I've flicked to sports pages on my phone to check for trade news, as his slightly hairy ass mechanically bobs away in front of me.

Four: sympathy. Or maybe grubbiness. When the deed is done, I notice that the actress is looking a little pained.

> Me: You didn't look as though you were having that much fun?
> Actress: It looked like I was in pain, right?
> Me: Well, in between, a few times.
> Actress: I, yeah, I was.
> Me: Yeah?
> Actress: But I, it's probably not going to be my best scene but . . .
> Me: Been working too much lately?
> Actress: Not too much, just yesterday was, the guy was huge and
> I've never, ever even, like, seen something that big, so [*sighs*], it
> kinda hurt. Still hurts today.

She gets dressed and instantly becomes incredibly alluring. Strange to have barely stirred while seeing her naked and penetrated, only to find her strikingly sexy the moment she's covered up. A porn set is an odd place to wonder whether the hijab is a genius idea; that nothing is sexier than what's left to the imagination.

The director, winding up his camera cable, has the battle-worn shrug of a man who sees naive exuberance turn sour every week.

"They think it's going to be fun and games. People don't realize that you come to porn, it's work. You're not just having sex with good-looking dudes or guys having sex with good-looking chicks. It's work. And they don't realize it's not that much money. So, you know, for a girl to make a decent living, she's got to do, like, eighty to a hundred scenes in a year. It's a lot of scenes, it's a lot of [*makes sex motions with his fingers*]. You do that for a while, your finger starts hurting [*laughs*] so you can imagine."

I find the male actor—a good-looking bugger with more than a hint of the French soccer player David Ginola—by his motorbike, outside the nondescript suburban house they've been filming in. I decide not to bring up the fact that he was cast today, in part, because his unthreatening girth was unlikely to exacerbate the situation. Instead, we chat about the almost total lack of condoms on porn sets these days.

"Because nobody wants it," he says. "It's not me. If that would be my call, my decision, I would put a condom on every single shoot, because I think the health of people is very important. But then, the shoot doesn't work that way. They don't care about our health. All they care about is making money, and they care about the girls looking good, and they care about the movie looking good, and they care about people buying movies."

And with that, he's onto his Kawasaki and off into the hills of northwest Los Angeles—an enclave that produces some 70 percent of the world's porn. By the standards of what else is being churned out in the other studios and rented houses around here, it was a pretty tame day's work.[1]

WHEN PORN WAS PORN

I embraced porn from a precocious age. At about ten or eleven, I would head down to WH Smith's newspaper store in Altrincham to buy a copy of the *Sun*, then whisk its clandestine Page 3 nipplefest home inside a copy of the *Manchester Evening News*. Such were the innovative lengths a young almost-hormonal boy had to go to in his quest for a nipple in the 1980s. Bizarrely, like some sort of prepubescent garage mechanic, I took to pinning up the topless photos of glamour models Sam Fox and Linda Lusardi on my wall amid the Man City team posters, which at least ensured no friends ever passed up the chance to come over to my house. To my parents' relief, and my friends' disappointment, I soon drifted apart from Linda and Sam. The teen years were fairly barren yet rudimentary on the porn front. The odd porno mag got passed around school—a crumpled page of one was kept in my secret drawer, featuring a semiclad woman lying on a snooker table, beneath the thrilling words "Can I lick your balls?"—and after band practice, someone once stuck on a VHS video that lasted about as long as the band itself.

At college, I graduated to crowding around a PC as a smutty picture tantalizingly revealed itself pixel by pixel, during which time you could pop the kettle on and finish off that week's Reformation coursework. Like most of my generation, I entered adulthood as a young man who'd seen boob, bum, some bush, and the odd simulated sex scene: no actual penetration, and anal sex was so distant as to be from another planet. A diet of words and photos—leaving what actual intercourse would look like as something for the imagination to piece together. There were no visual, visceral *expectations* for what sex should be like; you were left to discover that for yourself with an actual human during freshman term.

Apart from the few snatched minutes of imported German video, it was probably not that much more revealing than anything previous generations of schoolboys had managed to see. Like the poor Eton pupil—"son of the colonel in the army, a brilliant lad"—who, in the words of the former head of the Metropolitan Police in 1910, "had been reduced to driveling imbecility as the result of secret sin, induced by the sight of an obscene photograph exhibited by a scoundrel whom he met in a railway train. I had the satisfaction of hunting the villain down and of procuring him a long sentence of penal servitude."[2] Quite what the photograph was, the copper never says, but he was addressing a purity rally of Corn Flakes–munchers, so it was probably nothing more than a copy of *Edwardian Babes*.

It's hardly surprising that seventeenth-century serial groper Samuel Pepys managed to avail himself of the popular imported French pornography that was doing the rounds in London. Having come across a copy of a sex manual, *L'Escholle des Filles*, in a bookshop, he declared it "the most bawdy, lewd book" he'd ever seen—in fact he was "ashamed of reading in it." So ashamed that he returned later to buy a copy—in a plain binding—just to "inform himself of the villainy of the world." And he really managed to overcome that shame when he skipped church the next day to leaf through the book, with its crude drawings of the wheelbarrow position and encouragements to "Finger yield a Wench." All too much for Pepys, who wrote in his pseudo-Spanish, "it did hazer my prick stand all the while," leading to "una vez to decharger."[3] He then burned the book—the 1688 equivalent of shutting the laptop in hasty shame.

Pepys would never make it to church, that young Etonian never recover from his driveling imbecility, if they were teleported in front of a computer today. In a Pepys-like commitment to research, I've clicked onto YouPorn to discover which are the most popular videos streaming today. Today's top six:

Slutty MILF Takes Huge Black Cock POV
Cute Brunette Fucks in Public for Extra Cash
Dirty Girl Shelby Visits a Local Gloryhole to Give Blowjobs to
  Strangers and Swallows Their Cum
Alexis Adams Receives Explosion of Cum on Her Pretty Face
New Face Destiny Love Wants Anal for the First Time
Extreme Teen Fist Fucking Penetrations

Just some of the coyly titled clips drawing some 3 million users a day to this one site[4]—YouPorn claims to have 100 million page views per day[5]—for their average of eight minutes and thirty-six seconds of pleasure.[6] You certainly couldn't fault them under the Trade Descriptions Act; the clips do what they say on the label, though the MILF did look young to be a mother (maybe it's a sign of aging, that policemen and MILFs seem way too fresh-faced these days), and if we're being honest, Destiny Love, I suspect someone's fibbing about this being the loss of your anal virginity.

Fisting, facials, double penetration, glory-hole blowjobs in full HD close-up—we barely bat an eyelid. Oh, that's just what's clogging up 30 percent of the internet's bandwidth.[7] The barriers to seeing this sort of hardcore action used to be suitably off-putting: having to actually walk into a sex shop on a commercial street, or entering your credit card details online. There was a natural selection to this: only the most dedicated deviant—a true connoisseur of filth—would risk stumbling out of a grubby sex shop clutching a brown paper bag. Hardcore was the preserve of the real minority. And the 7 million monthly circulation of a *Playboy* or *Penthouse* during their 1970s "Pubic Wars"[8] was the high-water mark of soft-core porn. Mainstream today—just a free click away, zero entry barriers—is an all-you-can-gorge buffet of gynecological-grade wank-size bites. Context-free cocks, anuses, vaginas, and mouths colliding in every permutation, with no semblance of a storyline or plot to build appetite or cleanse the palate. With barely any meaningful regulation controlling what's being dished up in that eight minutes of onanism.

One of the few porn producers to have fallen foul of the law is Max Hardcore. "I really enjoy my work," he said, "and I also, in some way, enjoy pushing the limits and rubbing their faces in it and saying, 'Yes, I can do that.'"[9] *What* was being rubbed into faces became too much for the Justice Department. His extreme videos, with a penchant for aggression, urination, and fisting, landed him in a federal jail for two and a half years in 2009. I caught up with a British actress who had starred in his films—Barbii Bucxxx—back home from LA, on a soulless suburb up north in England. She described him as a "total psycho"—with peculiar dietary demands for his costars.

"He makes the girls eat beforehand a sort of breakfast roll with meat and the flat sausage and the egg, 'cause the egg's quite chunky and it doesn't solidify in your stomach. So he gets you to eat something that will end up coming out chunky." Vomit porn—if ever there was a metaphor for gorging gone too far.

To see just how much this on-tap, anything-goes porn makes previous generations look like a dusty VHS tape with a curled-up sticker, I spoke to Sharon Mitchell, an adult star from the seventies and eighties who went on to run a sexual health clinic in LA dedicated to porn performers.

"If I were a young girl today, there would be no way that I would work now. When I started, there were only thirty actors and actresses, and we all knew each other, and we were basically all out of work or, you know, legitimate actors and actresses not working enough, and it was very communal, very familial. It was the height of the sexual revolution, and it was fun being a rebel. That actually meant something," she says. "But now you can't pick your partner, you oftentimes can't use a condom, they don't pay remotely anything near to what they used to pay, and the amount of exploitation is incredible with the internet and everything."

Sharon starred when porn was porn: soft music, pizza delivery guys with awkward lines to deliver, and innocent-sounding titles like *Dial "P" for Pleasure*, *Wild in the Sheets*, and *Teacher's Favorite Pet*. A striking woman in her fifties, with a short, dark bob and New Jersey accent, she spent more than a decade trying to keep performers healthy while the industry started "getting more and more extreme."

"This is the world I lived in every day. You know, people asked, 'Can this guy ejaculate on a bare eyeball—is that OK with you? How many chopsticks can I safely insert in someone's ass?' And I thought to myself,

Hmm, now in what part of school, medical or psychological school, would I have learned how many fucking chopsticks it would take? So I said, 'I'm not sure, but just always insert from the middle and make sure that they're plastic and sterile.' I mean, you know, I never knew what I was going to hear every day. I never knew, but I can tell you short of driving a train up someone's ass, it's definitely getting more extreme."

YES, YES, YES. NO.

Porn is way more prevalent and extreme than ever before. So what? Can't this, in some way, be a good thing for men? We're now free to indulge and celebrate our true sexual tastes, however obscure or extreme they might be. We've shaken off the lingering, religious-fueled morality that has been forced down our throats for centuries, which denied man's true sexual nature. Merely picking up where the ancient Greeks left off, with their porny pottery, such as the drinking cup from around 510 BCE, attributed to Pedieus Painter, which graphically depicts a woman being spit-roasted by two men, while the older of the two hits her with a sandal.[10] And we are able to harness the power of porn to inject some inspiration and variety into flagging sex lives to keep relationships afloat.

Hmm. So why did I come back from the valleys of LA feeling like I needed to take a long shower (not of the Max Hardcore variety)? Why do I wish I'd never clicked onto an internet porn site—and if there was an "erase all images from the mind" button, I'd gladly send the lot to the hippocampic trash? Maybe some of this self-reproach stems from the whiff of that lingering moral judgment still hanging in the ether from centuries of sexually repressive "masturbation is self-pollution" teaching, reinforced, latterly, by the obscenity (note the inherently judgmental) laws.

Despite a majority of men watching porn—one study more reliable than most found that 68 percent of young adult men used porn at least once a week[11]—similar numbers (around 65 percent of males) see viewing adult content as morally unacceptable.[12] The left hand does know what the right is doing, but it can't wait to shut the laptop in shame.

This private double standard feeds a public sanctimoniousness. In 2015, four British judges lost their positions for viewing porn on work computers, a "wholly unacceptable conduct for a judicial office-holder," concluded the disciplinary inquiry.[13] Stripped of their livelihoods, after decades of collective public service, and humiliatingly publicly named. Careers ruined, for what? For taking a few minutes out from the working day, in the privacy of their chambers, to view some perfectly legal porn. Something that, as anyone who has worked from home can testify, can actually be an *aide à la concentration*. One of the judges said he was suffering from "severe and undiagnosed depression" at the time; while not therapy covered by most insurance, porn can temporarily click you out of feeling numb—it's understandable why he might have strayed onto an adult site. Lesser punishments than dismissal have been handed out for judges who have seemingly fallen asleep during rape trials.[14] And it was a minor misdemeanor compared to the actual bodily discharge of one old judge who apparently became so excited when sentencing someone to be hanged that he used to ejaculate in court; according to his clerk, a fresh pair of trousers had to be brought to court for death-sentencing occasions.[15] Yet four men's careers and reputations have been trashed, with all the personal and family fallout that follows, for partaking in something more mainstream than watching football. Of course, you can't go around watching porn on an office computer when you're at work; it was nuts and showed serious technological and workplace naiveté. But the scale of the punishment had the distinct stench of excessive public prurience. Surely a smack on the offending wrists would have done the job.

I really don't think the sanctimonious disciplining of m'lewds, the judges had any bearing on my post-LA aversion to porn. Not for someone raised under the watchful eye of Sam and Lucinda, for whom *Portnoy's*

Complaint was the set text of adolescence. Why I took issue with porn—and perhaps why so many who regularly use adult content will still class it as morally unacceptable—is that deep down we know it's just not good for us. And the more you peel back the façade, like peering into the kitchen of a fast-food restaurant, the less savory it seems.

Had I been writing this after my graduation, I'd have mounted a basic defense for porn. The monthly delivery of *High Society* or *Hustler* was no worse than having the occasional Big Mac, pint, or cig—the odd vice in moderation adds to the spice of life—and nor will a few smutty pictures or a couple of minutes of an actress shouting "*Schnell, schnell, wunderbar!*" lead to mass loss of respect for women. But today's porn truly is a different beast: it's weapons grade.*

And it has proliferated beyond control, to be on-tap with one tap to anyone with even the vaguely smartest of phones.

For the man who is committed to making a go of monogamy and working to maintain sexual attraction past that initial lusty phase, just about the last thing he needs is to be carrying around a limitless supply of hard-core sex scenes in his pocket. Scenes filled with women whose bodies bear little resemblance to ordinary anatomical reality, making noises that are only heard elsewhere for a fortnight during Wimbledon, seemingly gleefully taking part in acts that are somewhat unlikely to be a staple on the menu of relationship sex. When compared to that familiar once-a-week-ish sex, how can this not breed some seed of sexual dissatisfaction? Especially when this lurid mass of HD flesh is landing on highly susceptible gray matter: the male brain.

Men are sexually visual animals. Emory University psychologists have found that the emotion control center of the brain, the amygdala, shows significantly higher levels of activation in males viewing sexual visual stimuli than females viewing the same images.[16] Porn short-circuits to a man's

---

*Nor can it be seen as resuming ancient Greek business. As Alain de Botton says, their smutty pottery has to be viewed in the context of seeing sex itself as "a moment to celebrate the god-like perfection of our bodily selves"—with the body itself "an indication of inner virtue." Not something that tends to be routinely conveyed on xHamster.

emotional HQ. Indeed, we are so visually driven that women may have evolved pendulous breasts once hominids began walking upright just to keep us happy, replicating the fatty buttock deposits we'd been lovingly gazing at when knuckle-walking.[17] Surely the slowest sext response ever:

"Send me a photo of your fatty deposits—I miss them."
"Hold on. Let me evolve a new pair."

Monkey sees, then he wants to do. That a thirty-year-old heterosexual British man in 2010 was three times more likely (from 6 to 18 percent) to have had anal sex in the last twelve months than if he'd been born twenty years earlier—with 50 percent of the 2010 men reporting having ever tried it[18]—must be a direct link to the sheer prevalence of anal sex in porn. Once the niche preserve of the brown paper bag, anal sex has moved to the mainstream; it's tempting to feel short-changed when it doesn't make a cameo in a scene. An analysis of 10,000 porn stars shows 62 percent of actresses have done anal, while 39 percent have performed simultaneous anal and vaginal double penetration.[19]

Yet let's not slip into knee-jerk puritanism. Porn's impact is far from black and white. That more (straight) adults are trying and having anal sex could be seen as porn blowing off the cobwebs of centuries of damnation—late Medieval Christian clerics called for anal sex to be punished by three years of fasting[20]—giving people permission to try a bit of what they fancy. Likewise, there's no mystery anymore about what gets a man's amygdala going. The joy of receiving a sext—a bespoke porny photo—is on a par with seeing your team win the league in overtime after a forty-four-year barren patch. Women may wonder why a disembodied photo of their crotch can bring as much pleasure as a beautiful goal or long bomb caught in the end zone, but don't ask me—ask the almond-shaped set of neurons in the medial temporal lobe.

Our sex lives may have been spiced up—and phones clogged up—but our susceptible minds have been filled with expectations and images of sex that are wildly unrealistic. Buggering around with the expectations of something as core to the human condition as sex and intimacy is bound to end in tears. The relationship charity Relate reports a "huge increase" in online-driven compulsive sexual behavior among men,[21] porn seems to be increasingly cited as a factor in divorce,[22] and studies suggest the use of explicit content is associated with higher-risk sexual behavior and lower sexual satisfaction.[23]

Hopefully, most men can mentally brush off what they've viewed. But for some, it is a desensitizing escalator: once vaginal, anal, and both at once become a bit *So what?* the brain demands ever more explicit, taboo, or unusual stimulation. Porn not just reflecting tastes but creating new ones, seared on the visual memory, which never would have existed in the first place. Tastes that are further and further away from reality.

I once spent a morning with a censor at the British Board of Film Classification who was vetting films for their R18 listing—the strictest category, only available in sex shops (before it all gets pirated online anyway). We both kept admirably straight faces while watching a film in which a guy took a woman into the kitchen and used some sort of metal contraption to clamp open her vagina before mixing inside her all the ingredients for an omelet—which then plopped into a frying pan when she stood up. Despite my concerns over the salmonella risk from the raw eggs, the film was given the go-ahead. If I were erasing my porn memory, this would be the first file in the "Delete" queue. But if egg-based porn happens to be the thing that really gets you going, I suspect that's going to be a difficult one to broach with the missus after doing the dishes. (While not specifically the *oeuf oeuvre*, I have talked to women whose partners could only perform in bed while simultaneously watching a specific genre of porn.)

I left the viewing, blinking into the midday sun of Soho Square, with diminished appetite—but grateful that my neural pathways had long since been formed. What on earth will be the long-term impact on kids being brought up in an era where seriously hard-core porn is so prevalent: what will they come to expect as normal? What image of women is being fixed in boys' minds? Already, one in ten twelve- to thirteen-year-olds fears they are addicted to porn, the children's charity NSPCC has found.[24]

A young man whose six-year porn addiction started when he was fifteen admitted, "I couldn't get erections anymore with real women when I tried because I'd watched so much porn. It wasn't exciting anymore to be with a real woman." That desensitizing escalator kicked in. "You watch things you really wouldn't ever watch. . . . I was watching things that disturbed me, that weren't in keeping with what I knew my sexuality was, things like transsexual porn and gay porn."[25]

And what might be experimental or playful for an adult takes on a sinister—and pressurized—hue when acted out by young people. Like sexting. A social worker told me about some eleven- to thirteen-year-old boys who had formed a social media group where they'd upload intimate "conquest" photos of girls and detail what each was willing to do.

Boys exposed to porn are not just growing up with unrealistic impressions of women's appearances; it's also feeding the self-doubt about what *they* should look like. Aware of the rising numbers of boys lacking self-esteem around body image, I can't imagine porn is anything but a corrosive factor among others including advertising and social media. A US pediatric study found that nearly 18 percent of adolescent boys were "extremely concerned with their weight and physique." The report noted that in their desire to look more muscular, young men are as likely to abuse growth hormones and steroids as young women are to become bulimic to look thinner. "Relatively little is known about eating disorders among males," it concluded.[26]

When young men do get around to using the moves they've been taught online, they might get a rude awakening. Following the porn curriculum to elicit center-court shrieking from women might well lead to a backhand return. "I will say that some of the younger clients that I see, I call them Duracell Bunnies. These are guys who watch a steady diet of porn," says Laura, our Irish escort. "You can tell the minute they walk through the door. These are the ones who think good sex is about how long you can pound away for, and of course it's not. The ones who think if they lightly slap your cheek, it's highly erotic. So they get told very quickly to get back in their box and behave themselves."

So porn is not ideal for our visually suggestive brains, our minds trying to grapple with intimacy and enduring attraction, how we look at our own bodies, and, if we allow any postcome clarity to creep in, our consciences. I'd love to be able to say that after weeks of observing the porn business up close I left feeling that I'd been witnessing female empowerment in action: eyes-open sassy women choosing to make good money on their own terms. However, virtually every actress I met seemed to have a damaging backstory: substance dependency, an exploitative boyfriend who'd led them into the business, or a history of abuse. One of the male actors I talked to on set told me the saying about the actresses was "Mommy didn't love them enough, Daddy loved them too much." He didn't buy into the notion that he'd just been aiding female empowerment. "I've had to work with girls that before a scene were crying in the bathroom, and that's not easy, you know. And there is probably more of that than there are the sexually liberated girls." Female porn stars last an average of eighteen months in the business before quitting. (It might well be a more positive and maybe liberating experience to appear in the genre of films directed by, and aimed at, women, rather than just those created for base male instant gratification.)

The one seeming exception to these dark undertones came in the blonde, buxom, five-foot-ten vision of Wigan loveliness, Nikki Jayne—who'd swapped a call center in Greater Manchester for becoming the latest porn starlet sensation in LA. If my life were to flash before me, alongside the singing grannies—though hopefully not abutting each other in the flashback—would be the afternoon I spent Rollerblading with Nikki down Venice Beach and her having to catch me as I semi-on-purpose kept losing my balance. I still see that afternoon in slo-mo. Nikki—real name Samantha—was a smart, funny, no-nonsense Northerner, who appeared to come from a perfectly nice family. So why was she now in LA doing a job where the first day at work entailed DP?

"I do like to be independent; it's not just money, it's also, you know, the sex industry's a massive, massive industry, and without actually being in the industry, how am I going to know the industry? Like I want to get into the producing side of it, I want to be on the other side of the camera, not in front of the camera. I mean, I'm not totally dumb, I know that us porn girls, we're just guinea pigs for the people at the top, for the agents and this and that."

Her agent did seem to be on the controlling side—later angrily barging in to break up an interview I was doing with her and lead her away. I, of course, fell for the male delusion of thinking I could "save" her—porn-star *Pretty Woman*—that she was talented enough to be doing something different, and called my agent to see if he'd represent her for daytime TV projects. He told me to have a cold shower. She went off to prep for something anatomically challenging.

While the industry might seem to be damaging to often already-damaged women, it wasn't entirely a bed of roses for the male performers either. I didn't feel this to the point of having any actual sympathy, or equal psychological concern, for the guys who get paid to have sex with porn stars for a living. But it was more a realization that it's actually quite a thankless job. The male stars are no more than hired, interchangeable appendages, who are way down the pecking order on set. They get a fraction of what the women earn, for handling—the men say—most of the pressure.

"It really is all about the guy," reflects veteran actor Randy Spears, one of only a couple of male porn stars who have any job security. "I mean, if the tool isn't working properly, you're not building a house, you know. That's for sure." We are sitting by the pool of a rented house, high up in the valley, after Randy has just finished a scene for Wicked films, the only company in town that insists on condoms. "I just don't want to get sick. Our business has grown so much and it's gotten so big, you don't have control anymore . . . and I care about my health. I think our entire business ought to be condom[-based]."

The pressure to make sure that the tool is working properly means that "almost everybody's on Viagra," says Alan, an introspective, handsome actor I met as he was getting ready to perform on another set with two blondes. "People will sometimes try to say that they don't take it, but, I mean, I think I've met like probably two or three who don't take it. You could be way into the girl too, but, like, just given the circumstances, it's pretty much a necessity. To establish a real connection is difficult," he explains.

"I have worked for different companies who want some extreme stuff, so I do my best to give it to them. Like she puked on me, and I was kind of dazed, and I looked over at the director because I had no idea if that's what he wanted. I knew that it was an extreme thing, but he was, like, keep going, you know, so . . . "

I ask Alan if he feels this industry has changed him. "Certainly, most certainly. In some ways for the better, in some ways for the worse. I grew up with Christianity—with religious guilt and whatever. And this has helped me get over it to a certain extent, especially if you do get to work with some girls who are just genuinely sexually liberated and just love sex." (Though *he* was the guy who said there weren't many of this liberated sort around.)

He told me on the way out that Viagra was wearing off for some of the guys, who were now injecting erectile-inducing chemicals into the base of their penises before scenes. Apparently, one chap overcooked the injections and was rushed to ER when his penis began to turn black.

But poisoned penises paled in comparison to the most truly disturbing consequence of porn that I stumbled across—which is occurring in the least likely of places.

During a tour of Anabolic, one of the major porn producers, their CEO mentioned in passing that they get a lot of fan mail from Ghana. He dug out one of the letters, from a Ghanaian called Mark, which had a photo attached of a sweet young man with no shirt on, whose return address was care of his local church in Accra.

"The reason why I am writing to you this letter is that I want to be an American sex star and I need your help. This is my picture and my number is . . . I hope to hear from you as soon as possible."

A wannabe porn star in West Africa writing to a specific company in LA was simply mind-boggling. Just how pervasive—and pernicious—was this content being shot in Southern California? Mark was a man I had to meet.

TOO FAR

In the main market in the middle of Accra, globalization is going great guns. Amid the fruit and veggie and casual sportswear stalls, the finest in hard-core Western porn is openly on sale. It's plain to see, in the racks of DVDs, how Mark may have got a taste for the LA stuff. While the search for Mark went on, I headed to the north of the country, where the tentacles of porn have spread to the most incongruous of places. The village looked like something from a *National Geographic* photoshoot: barefoot kids, goats wandering around, mud huts with thatched roofs, no electricity. But the lack of power is no impediment to determined men. Once a month, they bring a generator to the village—and turn one of the mud huts into a pop-up porn cinema, screening those Western films. What turns this from the surreal to the deeply disturbing is that, culturally, the men in the village don't believe in masturbation. So after the screenings, younger boys are sent out to go and bring back girls for their aroused older brothers.

I talked to a sheepish group of those older boys, who were sitting on a ledge by a hut, one wearing an out-of-date replica Arsenal shirt. He says he has "sleepless nights thinking about having sex." Another chillingly reveals, "You'll be thinking about having sex, but you don't have a partner. So it sometimes prompts you to go to rape somebody, to rape a woman in order to satisfy your sexual desire."

On the other side of the dusty village, I talk to a group of fifteen or so women, each with colorful scarves wrapped around their foreheads, the odd one clutching a baby. The looks are solemn when I bring up the videos. Many have stories to tell about their husbands being affected by these foreign films—of men no longer being satisfied by sex with them. One says that since her husband began watching porn three years ago, her marriage of thirty years has been collapsing.

It is almost beyond belief that a film shot in a Los Angeles suburb can somehow cause women to be raped and marriages to end in an African village 7,000 miles away that's barely been touched by modernity.

Nor do the ramifications end there. With just that one studio committed to condoms, the overwhelming majority of porn emanating from LA depicts unsafe sex. For their target audiences in the United States or Europe, there should at least be some level of sex education. For their inadvertent audiences in Ghana, the same cannot be said—which leads to deadly consequences.

In Accra, I met Kofi and Frank, two men who had watched rather a lot of porn over the years but had never had any sex education. So instinctively, they copied what they saw on screen, complete with its lack of condom use. "They were not using condoms, so I was not using," says Frank. They are both now HIV-positive.

Kofi took me back to his tiny shack of a house to meet his family. His four-month-old baby girl sleeping on a mattress was born HIV-free, but he has infected his wife. She pins her illness on the porn he watched. And Kofi says he just copied what he saw: "white is right."

Ghana's AIDS commissioner told me the impact of porn had the potential to undermine the country's fight against HIV and the inroads they have been making, calling it a "time bomb."

In the center of Accra, I finally catch up with Mark, the young man who wrote to the porn studio asking to be a star. He says he spends half his money on porn DVDs, and "just had the feeling I should write and saw their contact address at the end of the movie." It also turns out that he is chronically shy, can barely look me in the eye—and is a virgin. Yet such is his faith in the Land of the Free (porn), he is genuinely expecting a letter back inviting him out to LA to become a porn star.

Back in Los Angeles—with no sign of Mark, alas—I wondered how the porn genie, with its consequences for men and women globally, could ever be rebottled; sexual satisfaction was hard enough before all this came along. I unrealistically mused that perhaps the big porn companies should dispatch their stars to Africa to front safe-sex campaigns or make bespoke films for that market. A little corporate responsibility from a multibillion-dollar industry. Porn is of course going nowhere near that bottle. If it's clearly here to stay, perhaps the onus on the industry should be to generate more "fair-trade" porn, where the performers have emotional background checks and input into what they do, and the scenes have more context and reality. And have films made specifically for teens, who are going to watch porn regardless. Indeed, a Danish (naturally) professor believes it's time to show and deconstruct porn in classrooms, instead of the usual sex education "where you roll a condom onto a cucumber."[27] In my own commitment to ethical porn—in the weeks following my immersion in the industry—I very nobly restricted my clicks to Nikki Jayne.

I did also wonder if my own view of porn had become too jaundiced by what I'd seen—the women made to vomit, the horrors in the Ghanaian village. Journalistically, one is naturally drawn to tales of addiction and extreme behavior: *man watches porn, and there are no consequences* isn't the greatest story to explore. Did I have too much of a downer on porn? So I went to hear from the godfather of porn—Larry Flynt, the *Hustler* publisher who took a man's right to see a close-up of a vagina to the US Supreme Court. At the top of his Beverly Hills tower, he rolled over the thick green carpet in his gold wheelchair and told me that even *he* had problems with today's porn. "It makes it more difficult to defend what we do—and I think on a moral and social level, it's wrong."

When Larry Flynt says porn has gone too far, it must be hard-core.

11
A JEALOUS ATHEIST

WHY BIGGER BEARDS = LONGER LIVES
AND BETTER SEX

Grown men are rolling around on the floor, clutching their bellies, howling with uncontrollable laughter. Others shake in their seats while tears stream down their faces. A man who looks like a real estate agent is bent double, emitting howls of high-pitched hyena shrieking. Just another Sunday service at a charismatic church in Concord, New Hampshire, a bright-white A-frame chapel filled with several hundred worshippers. Just a run-of-the-mill gathering when your creed is "holy laughter."

I'm beckoned onto the stage at the front of the church. The pastor hands me the mic. "No one here is feeling any element of depression? Any anxiety?" I ask gingerly.

Momentary pause. Then full-on hysteria engulfs the chapel. A man in his fifties, dressed in chinos and sports jacket, lies on his back like an upended bug, legs kicking in the air, grasping his chest. I ask a guy with the build of a well-fed NFL player what's so funny; he can't catch his breath to answer me. Others manically dance on the spot, flinging their arms heavenward.

To a cynical, atheistic Brit, it felt like the height of Bible-thumping bonkerness. More evidence that crazy Creationists are cut from a different cloth. A further sign that people will do anything to fit in, even if that entails being swept up into an infantile wave of nearly peeing your pants. I felt like an alien who'd landed on a different planet. But compared to all the men who have walked on this earth—and to those who are on it today—I was the odd one out in that church. I was the freak for not believing that there is some greater divine purpose for why we are here. I was the weirdo for not embracing some sort of ritual to show my love for a God up high. And, frankly, they did seem to be having one heck of a time. It looked more fun than spending a Sunday evening on the couch half-watching a box set, banally chatting with girls on Tinder who have nice cleavage shots but terrible grammar.

Despite having been brought up with a modicum of religion—the bar mitzvah, a semblance of keeping kosher, an oversize medicine cabinet—it was the stuff of tradition rather than faith. What was probably a teenage agnosticism, which allowed for a little mystery, has slowly morphed into an unblinkered atheism. A skeptical eye that sees religion as manmade to suit our needs—and a source of serious strife.

Indeed, the very idea of gods—rather than our preagricultural belief in everything being part of some interconnected natural spirit—was born when we gave up foraging to settle down as farmers. With all that new unpredictability on where dinner was coming from, we conjured up particular gods to pray to for good crops and healthy flocks. (Wheat planting the seed for modern religion: is there no end to its glutenous reach?)[1] Nor does it take more than a fleeting glance at any newspaper to be reminded of the horrors being committed in the name of religion, with religion itself seeming to confer an extra layer of zeal and conviction to conflicts and persecution against group outsiders. A source of terrible repression against women, gays, and people who speak out; a medieval bulwark against safe sex and sex ed; a bogus authority for rulers to use to maintain the status quo. Not to mention the centuries of sexually dysfunctional teaching that still guiltily lingers.

So what if we've always been believers? For three thousand years, right until the end of the nineteenth century, the medical establishment believed in the therapeutic benefits of bloodletting,[2] needlessly killing off countless people with this voodoo (maybe even the first US president, George Washington, who had up to seven pints of blood taken after waking up with a sore throat—and snuffed it within four days).[3] It's a sign of our enlightenment that the scales have fallen from man's eyes regarding this religious mumbo jumbo.

And men in particular aren't buying these biblical tales any more. Women in the US (65 percent) are much more likely than men (46 percent) to pray every day.[4] In countries across the world, the clear majority of self-declared atheists are men, whether it be in Ukraine, Portugal, Japan, Israel, Mexico, Sweden, or Holland.[5] Who knows exactly why men are more likely to believe that we just happen to be on this planet, and that's that. Maybe we're more rational, have less social or psychological need for faith, are less exposed to the religious paraphernalia that can come with bringing up kids, and even more willing to take the risk of gambling that there's no heaven or hell to curry favor for.[6]

Yes, on a rational level, I—and plenty of men—will find it hard to argue with Richard Dawkins that there's not much in the way of supporting evidence for the "God Hypothesis."[7] But no matter how much I might intellectually agree with Dawkins, I can't help feeling that he's a bit of a party pooper. I can't help wondering whether, in our rush to cynicism, we've been a bit hasty to chuck out all the trappings of religion. I guess I have a slight confession: I'm jealous of religious men.

MIX-AND-MATCH REASONS I WISH I WERE RELIGIOUS

- I'd be well and truly married by now. Overpickiness and high expectations would have been swatted aside by the need to create a godly union under the impatient eye of an interfering community.

- I'd have really gotten on with the procreating. I met a rabbi recently who wasn't that much older than I am but had eleven kids—so many that he couldn't recall all their names off the top of his head. Talk about my Selfless Gene dawdling in the slow lane. Going to a weekly religious service means you're likely to have an average of 2.5 kids compared to the 1.67 from heathen loins.[8]

- I'd live seven years longer. Going to a religious service once a week also seems to add seven years to the clock, Dr. Harold Koenig from the Center for Spirituality, Theology, and Health at Duke University Medical Center told me. Indeed, he has found that "religious involvement is related to better coping with stress and less depression, suicide, anxiety, and substance abuse."[9] You can really start to see why those guys were nearly wetting themselves in that church.

- Yarmulkes/turbans/keffiyeh/taqiyah and all manner of head-dresses nicely cover up any male-pattern baldness, while Buddhism goes for the much more egalitarian shaved head. The world religions appear to have really taken into consideration male paranoia about hair loss. Alas, this seems to be an oversight for Christianity. The medieval Catholic tonsure—shaving in a massive bald spot for that Friar Tuck look—was largely banned by the Vatican in 1972,[10] but the pope and the clergy are all right Jack with their skullcaps.

- Confession looks like awesome therapy.

- Prayer (especially Islamic) looks good for back posture and gets you off that sedentary office backside.

- I would have steered clear of the more damaging impact of "vices," at least in theory. So I'd have had no bad-drugs trip;

never would have watched porn (though surveys of the URLs of religious men might suggest otherwise[11]); and never found myself fainting into a bush outside a hospital after a hypochondria-induced STD check. Standing in the middle of central London with an imam on a Saturday night, as a group of Liverpool lads proudly present their cocks and ask if we know where they can get some cocaine, the softly spoken Muslim leader reflected, "We're seeing people enjoy themselves and having fun. What we're not seeing are the consequences of this. For instance, we won't see the breakup of a marriage because of some act of infidelity, the liver damage that might come from this sort of activity, or the abortion that is going to ensue from that one-night stand." And then we were accosted by a hen party with a giant inflatable penis.

- I'd have been forced by the Sabbath, if I were an observant Jew, to take a full day off each week and unplug from the phone. And there'd be none of that wallowing in the morning: straight up and out for prayer, with lashings of that cardiovascular-pleasing group singing.

- Fasting is great for cell regeneration and the immune system, as many an underfed lab mouse reaching its giddy fourth birthday can testify. Indeed, the simple diet of the Greek monks of Mount Athos—with their unprocessed food and intermittent fasting—is now the ultimate fad. As the *Daily Mail* breathlessly asked, "Is the Greek MONK diet the key to staying slim and youthful? [New plan] mirrors eating habits of the devout Orthodox priests of Mount Athos who live 10 YEARS longer than average."

- I would have felt less pressure to achieve in this life as I could always have another crack when reincarnated in another.

In among the bizarre and arcane rituals and rules of religion—donkey drivers should have sex with their wives once a week, dictates the Mishnah, the Jewish legal code, whereas it's just monthly if you drive a camel[12]— perhaps there are kernels of wisdom that have evolved to help us understand the human condition. Forcing us to observe religious festivals means that we spend time with family and community no matter how busy we might protest we are at work. Saying a prayer before you eat is the heart of mindfulness, ensuring that you take a moment from the multitasking to focus on the food before you. The Japanese who gather each year for Zen-inspired moon-viewing parties must put the daily navel-gazing on hold to take a good look upward—how often do we do that?—putting into humbling perspective our antlike existence in this solar system.[13]

Shortcuts, evolved over millennia, that mean you don't have to work out everything yourself. Like tapping into some fairly powerful software that can make life easier and maybe more enriching to run—not to mention less glitchy than the Atheism OS. Shortcuts to some fundamental states that perhaps all chime with what really makes men tick.

Like: *belonging*. This is maybe our greatest urge, driving men to put their lives on the line like nothing else. The need to be part of a tribe, to have an identity. I don't believe in a higher being and would wager that the Old Testament was probably written by a bunch of guys over a several-hundred-year period, yet I still don't eat pork, might fast on Yom Kippur, and, if I have a son, would entirely irrationally want his foreskin lopped off. Likewise, it makes little sense to care whether eleven overpaid young men half your age kick a ball into a net or carry a misshapen one into an end zone—and it's hard to muster the same enthusiasm for something that was all you thought about when you were eight—but I still get a rush of blood when my team scores, and I still won't wear the red of our archrival. (There's nothing quite as nervously emasculating as being caught up in a football conversation where the gaps in your knowledge or passion are being exposed; it's such a strange badge of manhood. It has a playground potency that can make grown men who don't have a team or interest in the game feel quite alienated.) You can overanalyze the need to belong till the cows come home—maybe it's an insurance policy that means others will defend you under attack—but I just accept that I have my tribes. They help tether me; for whatever reason, they are part of who I am, and bacon and eggs remains off the menu.

Like: *having a bigger boss to please.* Whose performance evaluation on Judgment Day has nothing to do with your career, status, or bank balance—and who actually loves you. Does having an alternative belief system mean that a religious person might feel less stressed after a shitty day at work because it's not the be-all and end-all compared to his or her higher goals, while said person can also to write off setbacks as part of some bigger plan? Giving them that extra nudge toward doing a life-affirming good deed for someone else?

Like: *realizing that unvarnished reality is not all it's cracked up to be.* Video looks more dramatic in slow-motion, photos come to life with filters, but watching too much news can make you sadder and more anxious.[14] Religion can take the edge off the reality that this is just a meaningless genetic food fight, can allow for a little wonder to exist in the world—the feeling before some killjoy explained that the wonder of a rainbow was down to some refractive process—and can re-create that childlike reassurance that we're being looked after, even if we don't understand what the cosmic adults are getting up to.

And (maybe) like: *providing some delineation of gender roles.* If religious rules have been written by men for men, as they appear to be to the nonbeliever, then it's no surprise that we tend to do rather well out of it (apart from the undersexed camel drivers). But amid the self-serving subjugation of female rights that still persists in many religious guises, does religion offer another model of how men and women can relate to each other, a different, more traditional set of roles that some might feel more comfortable with? I popped around to see the Orthodox rabbi who hosted my near-fight night,

Mendel Cohen, a bearded bundle of energy from Leeds: seven years younger than me, a foot shorter, but winning 5–0 on procreation. He and his fast-talking American wife, Chai, have an avowedly equal relationship—and she works part-time—yet, as she says, being equal doesn't mean being the same. "Because men and women have differences, we have different roles in the world, some of which can overlap, some of which can't." Chai talked about women bringing a natural calm and stability to a home, of being instinctive around children, though she absolutely defended a woman's right to work. As a member of the Chabad tradition, she's in the rare position of being able to observe the modern and supertraditional, mixing both with the professional London wives who attend their Saatchi synagogue and the ultra-Orthodox Hasidic (serious beards, furry hats, no sniff of feminism) families when she takes her kids to school.

"The ultra-Orthodox women are under a lot less stress. Their expectations for life are clear. Whereas at the synagogue we have a lot of young working moms who've had their first kid and are under so much pressure. *Should I go back to work full-time?—but then I'm not going to see my kid. Should I stay home? I can't do my job part-time, so I'm gonna have to work so that in ten years my job will still be available to me.* So they're always going back and forward about the choices they're making and whether they're correct, whereas ultra-Orthodox people don't have that. They're confident that how they're living their life is how they want it to be."

Then, as if the heavens were parting and a chink of divine light were suddenly filling a nondescript office in northwest London, the rabbi and his wife imparted a piece of wisdom of truly biblical portions: the secret of maintaining sexual chemistry in a long-term relationship. From the time the wife begins her period—and for the week after it has ended, which culminates in a ritual bath—there can be no sexual contact at all. So there is a span of around twelve days a month when sex is forbidden (and some choose no physical touching at all, with separate beds). Mendel explained this via the parable of the cake. If there's an unlimited supply of chocolate cake in the fridge, after gorging for a week, you get bored with it, become complacent, and then start craving marble cake. And then, men especially get bored of that and move on to cherry cake, etc. But if you know there's one cake, you savor the last piece and look forward to when the next delivery is coming on, say, the following Monday; your relationship with it becomes psychologically much more exciting. You only lust for what you don't have. It makes you feel that your wife is not always permitted to you, so it brings passion and excitement." Chai concurred that this all keeps complacency and staidness at bay, citing her craving for pizza during the eight days of Passover, when flour is outlawed: "Anything that's forbidden you want." Is this ancient commandment to separate once a month a genius insight into our sexual psyches?

Beyond the lifespan-enhancing diet, hairline camouflage, nonnegotiable family time, tribal identity, bedroom wisdom, and this whole befuddling existence having purpose rather than being entirely random, where I am truly jealous of religious people is their faith in what comes next. If there was a single moment that caused me to desperately want to believe—a day when religion crashed into my life—it came out of the blue when I was seven years old.

April 15, 1983. A regular day at primary school. It was a Friday, so that afternoon we'd walked—in pairs, holding hands on the sidewalk—to the local playing fields for games. It was the joint birthday of two boys in my class, John, my oldest friend, and James, so I guess that would have been celebrated at some point.

It had been a regular sort of week. My mom, Helen, hadn't been around. She'd been in the hospital for what I thought, or maybe had been told, was a cold. But it had been no big deal, and one of the kindly teachers had been dropping me home after school. (The woman I talked about before, whom my dad divorced when I was thirteen, was my stepmom.)

I was a regular kind of seven-year-old—living with my mom, dad, brother, and Claude the cat in a regular kind of house in Manchester. I loved them, messed around with friends, was crazy for soccer, and the only prize they could think to give me at Sunday school was for chutzpah.

That Friday, after driving me home from school, the teacher came inside my house with me. There I found my dad sitting at the bottom of the stairs, with the rabbi, who lived opposite, next to him. My dad lifted me onto his knee and said, "Mum has gone to heaven." There might have been a line too about God needing her. I remember my dad's eyes being bloodshot, but he kept it together. I don't think I really took it in. How can a seven-year-old comprehend that his mother has died? That he would never again see the woman he waved goodbye to from the landing the week before as she left the house in a beige overcoat to go to the hospital—an image I can still picture like a faded Polaroid. Whenever I see a kid of that age now, it just seems *so* young, way too young to take it in.

I'd had no inkling that she was ill. In retrospect, I can recall her spending a bit of time in bed, and I'd seen a pad that went in her bra to fill where a breast had been removed. But it had been a total thunderbolt from nowhere. I guess in those days there was no therapeutic thinking about how to soften the blow for children, to prepare them for their world imploding. Nor was there any counseling afterward. There was a funeral, which I didn't attend, and lots of women bringing around endless dishes of food, then back to school. I remember my first day back, sitting next to John, feeling very spaced out as I tried to catch up on the work that I'd missed. Life went on, but with an enormous emotional hole in it. Nine months later, my brother Mark had his bar mitzvah.

At least I'm blessed to have a sharp childhood memory and can remember being with her. Being on the back of her bicycle as we rode to school and my iced bun falling on the road. Running to her after putting the brake of my bike through my cheek. Staying in to play with her when it was snowing outside and I had a cold. The memories remain clear and cherished. That raw sense of loss faded into the background—something to think about on occasion rather than routinely—but it will always remain my most tender emotional spot. Just about the only thing that can make me cry is to summon up memories of my mum. I cannot bring myself to visit her grave in Manchester. Perhaps I'll feel differently when, hopefully, I have my own family—once the life cycle has fully revolved around to being a parent myself.

Many an hour has been spent in therapy trying to deduce what the impact of all this has been. Boy, how a therapist sits up in his chair when you throw in a maternal loss at some supposedly critical age in childhood development. And the earnest nodding goes into near-whiplash overdrive when you mention that three years later, when I was ten, my dad remarried, only for that to end in door-kicking divorce. So, yes, I seemed to have carelessly lost two people I called Mum by the age of twelve, and those can't be the ideal foundations for later commitment in life. What I can't fathom out is whether this "stuff" becomes hardwired in who you are, or whether once you bring it to the surface, through talking, you can break it down and start to shift it. It feels a bit of a cop-out to claim you're forever defined by what might have happened to you as a kid, but who knows what psychological legacy you're up against.

My brother and I both agree the experience fired us into a headlong hurry to make our mark. Years ago, I read an interview with the UK broadcaster Chris Evans whose father died, of cancer too, when he was thirteen. He said it was like a "starting gun" being fired; at such a young age you're suddenly confronted with mortality and know there's no time to waste. I read the words over and over. The penny dropped on why I had spent my teenage weekends precociously trying to get on air at Piccadilly Radio—exactly as Chris had done the decade before—and university years attempting to become the media baron of the three streets of St. Andrews. Meanwhile, my brother had passed his student time dangling in various abseil-based protests from the University of London Union, of which he was president.

But despite my mom's death being presented to me in religious terms—of her being called by God—it never pushed me toward religion. I used to play a game in my head of what would I do to get to see her again. Ridiculous measures, like, *Would I chop off my finger for an evening in her company?* So how beyond amazing it must be if you do have the conviction that there is an afterlife, that one day you will be with your lost loved ones again. Seeing my mum again, to have a hug from her, is probably the thing my soul most craves. The idea that this could actually happen is too immense to even begin to comprehend. Yet, hand on heart, as much as every fiber of my being might will its possibility, I just can't believe this will one day happen. I just don't have the faith in an afterlife or God. Why not?

DNA-WOL

On its most basic level, I just don't "feel" it—whatever that feeling is. Religious people talk about a *love* for Jesus or God. Could it be like those first throes of a relationship when you feel a little high, full of boundless certainty and flushed with oxytocin rushes that make you want to bore everyone with how great you feel? Does thinking about Jesus, say, bring about the same sort of feel-good flushes, which you just have to share? At a gathering of religious people—or a political rally these days—it does sometimes look like someone has dropped an oxytocin bomb, such is the unnerving level of conviction and zeal. Was the laughter church a roomful of adults drunk on love? In a Church of England service, it's perhaps more of a low-key, shoe-staring *I think I'm rather fond of you* love. Could the fact that I've never felt any approximation of this be because I—along with other agnostics and atheists—just don't have the right genes?

Studies of identical twins, including those who were brought up apart, suggest that genes contribute about 40 percent of the variability in a person's religiousness. And that as we get older, genes become more important in determining how religious we are, while environmental factors, such as how we were raised, tail off. One geneticist has, not without controversy, specifically identified a version of the VMAT2 gene that is more prevalent in "spiritual" people, who tangibly feel a connection to the universe. This "God gene" produces greater levels of dopamine in believers, making it feel good and rewarding to believe in God.[15] Could it possibly be that part of the reason I don't believe in a divine being lies in the particular version of the VMAT2 gene I have on my chromosome 10?

All of which comes back to faith as being inspired by a feeling, rather than necessarily arriving at belief through logical analysis. The only religion that appears to make any logical sense to me is Buddhism, which seems to get a good handle on human nature—believing that our constant cravings make us miserable—doesn't rely on a creator figure, and goes big on the meditation. I guess I should become a JuBu—culturally Jewish, spiritually Buddhist—if someone could do the honors of bringing it to England.

One note I would add, though, is that I know *my* feelings aren't always accurate when they are at their most negative. When I'm down, it's easier to draw the wrong conclusions about people—who, say, aren't ignoring you but are in fact just busy—or misread situations. So maybe, just maybe, we miserable atheists with our lower-dose dopamine are on too much of a divine downer to read the world as it really is and aren't picking up on a spiritual frequency that's out there. God knows.

It was definitely easier to draw clearer and consistent conclusions about porn than existential purpose and genetic disposition. In search of one final attempt at getting another wafer's crumb of insight into what makes a man believe, I went to talk God with someone who, of the people I know, strikes me as one of the least likely to be religious.

A. A.—Adrian—Gill. Probably Britain's most renowned and non-prisoner-taking television and restaurant critic. The one you *really* don't want to have been paying close attention when one of your less-than-illustrious shows airs. Someone who deconstructs narratives—and scythes through hoodwinkery—for a living.

Yet, each night, he and his young son and daughter say their prayers together. Adrian believes.

Not that his critical faculties have rolled over in the face of the Good News.

"I'm a very doubting Christian, and I spend most of my time as a Christian doubting things and being incredulous. I don't believe the Bible is remotely literal, I don't think it's a history of things that happened as they say. I think it was written by people who were trying to understand something that is innately not understandable. But I do think there was somebody called Jesus and he was probably special—and he was innately good."

When I mentioned to a media friend that I was off to talk God with Gill, they mumbled, "*Well, he was an alcoholic, you know.*" Like Death Row inmates, alcoholics have new-follower form; our all-knowing cynicism isn't surprised when the bottle and Bible are gripped by the same hand. Gill heads this off before I even raise it.

"I was brought up an atheist—my father was a card-carrying atheist. . . . I never had a revelation, I haven't heard voices or seen visions, there's not a *thing*. I am a recovering alcoholic and drug addict, and people often associate that with coming to God. But actually, I had a belief in God before I ever got sober or clean. So it wasn't that. It was a slow understanding/belief/faith—a slow growing into faith, just this sense that I wasn't alone in the world."

Could this faith have grown because the genetic material was fertile?

"I've been manipulating my dopamine levels consistently and very effectively . . . and the sense of belief, of faith, is nothing like giving yourself a rush or a hit of a drug. Not for me; it may be for some people."

When I see those overexuberant Americans rolling around the church floor, or ultra-Orthodox Hasidics shuffling away at the Western Wall, their faith is less surprising, as they are somehow *other*. What I find more intriguing is how someone of a familiar, skeptical British disposition arrives at not feeling alone in the world. What *is* this feeling that inspires faith?

"It's not a physical sensation—it's a sort of understanding," he says. "There are long periods where what you have is almost overwhelming doubt or distance. You feel yourself quite distant from it. That it's a very faint conversation that's happening three doors down. And there are other times when it's absolutely a hand on your shoulder," he says.

"So within the rational doubt, there are moments of intense faith and sometimes they're just flashes. They're just pinpricks. Moments of trust, of understanding, of something of a feeling. It isn't a thing I can describe as anything other than faith. And describing faith to someone who doesn't have faith is difficult—because it's not like anything else."

We got cake and pizza metaphors from the rabbi and his wife—don't let the Christians down now.

"Somebody said a belief in God is like being a child underneath a table and all you see is the tablecloth; and you just assume that on the table there is this incredible meal set. But all you see is the edge of the tablecloth." And: "It's like holding a string that disappears up into the clouds, and every so often there's a little tug on the string—but you don't know what's tugging it, and you don't know why."

As my string envy and I prepared to go, leaving Adrian to skewer a pretentious fish restaurant, I wondered whether any Christian-fueled guilt ever encroached when he was penning a scathing review.

"That somehow having a faith would lead you toward being a kindly liar? . . . I don't see that." (Adrian sadly died of cancer not too long after I spoke to him.)

GOOD APPLES

I don't wake up each morning thinking, *Gosh, if only the world were a more religious place.* What the Middle East could *really* do with right now is just a bit more religion. If only Africa had a few *more* people discouraging condom use. And I'm just *so* relieved Bush and Blair were men of such iron religious conviction when mulling what to do with Iraq. Nor do I personally yearn to grow my beard to food-catching, flight-missing proportions, swing a chicken around my head once a year (transferring bad deeds to the poultry), or renounce masturbation (Onan was killed in Genesis for his seed-spilling sins).

I don't have some idealized notion of religion. When I do end up in a church or synagogue, it's a battle against boredom and retro fidgeting. Yet I am slightly torn. On a terribly simplistic level, I do think men who have religion are—in some ways—lucky buggers. The alchemy of on-tap community, the framework of rules, and the inner feelings of faith and purpose seem to produce enough benefits to make people live longer and have more stable mental health. Which is all very nice for believers, whose VMAT2 deserves a pat on the back.

But for us men who, in greater numbers than ever before, are left distinctly cold by religion, is there anything we can take from this? Is there something even an atheist can copy and paste from this Religion OS before sending it all to the trash?

Short of inducing a see-the-light moment—though geneticists can have a pop at a pill for that once they've worked out how to stop the promiscuous meadow vole from getting its leg over—I'd say the most potentially fertile territory lies in the rituals. To not throw the baby out with the baptism water and see which of the more enlightened rituals that are buried in each religion might still have meaning regardless of faith—from small acts of mindfulness that snap us out of our day-to-day heads, to the occasions that bring us together and give primacy to family, food, and music. (In addition to yoga, meditation, and mindfulness, I'm sure there are more practices that we can mine from the East too.)

Religious rules and rituals are a bit like morals, which, as Bukowski wrote, "were restrictive, but they *were* grounded on human experience down through the centuries. Some morals tended to keep people slaves in factories, in churches and true to the State. Other morals simply made good sense. It was like a garden filled with poisoned fruit and good fruit. You had to know which to pick and eat, which to leave alone."[16]

With creative thinking, these arcane religious rites that have stood the test of time can even be refashioned to have modern meaning. Some entirely secular US friends, for example, have done just that with the Jewish Sabbath—that traditional mandated day of rest that starts just before sunset on Friday and ends when three stars appear in the sky on Saturday evening, during which time Orthodox Jews are forbidden from using electricity, traveling, and anything approximating work. The group, Reboot, has taken the essence of this day of rest but given it a spin that's relevant to how we live today. Their Sabbath Manifesto suggests that on one day a week—and for an annual national Day of Unplugging to bring a real sense of scale—we could:

1. Avoid technology.
2. Connect with loved ones.
3. Nurture our health.
4. Get outside.
5. Avoid commerce.
6. Light candles.
7. Drink wine.
8. Eat bread.
9. Find silence.
10. Give back.

What's coyly buried in the second principle is that this "connection" can be to make sweet love to your partner—which is traditionally seen as a holy activity for the Sabbath. Some scholars have suggested that the age-old Sabbath meal of chicken soup, with its matzo balls suggestively bobbing around, is actually an aphrodisiac to warm up for the big connection.[17] It's always struck me more as an elephant-grade sedative that leaves tie-stained men dribbling on the couch before the strudel is even served.

In terms of life guidance, religion has thrown up some real stinkers over the years—perhaps nothing tops old Origen and his early Christian friends removing their own testes to be more chaste.[18] But to separate the wheat from the repressive chaff, there are some nuggets of wisdom in among it all. And across the disparate religions, there are common insights on how men, in particular, should live—which resonate with other areas of masculinity we've been looking at. Having some rite of passage that marks boys' transition to manhood. Celebrating the wisdom of elders, not marginalizing old people. Carving out dedicated space for men to spend time together, which could prompt discussion of some fairly meaty stuff beyond the usual conversational diet of football scores and who's going to make the playoffs. Bringing a bizarre but maybe strangely wise understanding to what maintains sexual chemistry in a relationship, whether that be around imagination-driven visual modesty or a monthly physical separation to build anticipation. Underpinning all of this, religions recognize that men and women can't be lumped together as one amorphous mass.

And lo, my confession endeth.

And, in return for this atheist respect, don't be shy one day with the seventy-two virgins/eternal nirvana/paradise tickets (plus one)—and maybe send down some of the other VMAT2 genes in the meantime.

12
PATERNITY TEST

TRYING TO BE A GOOD DAD AND NOT-SO-BAD LAD

In 1960, a young expectant father wanted to be with his wife when she was giving birth. The twenty-three-year-old Humboldt State University student accompanied his partner to their local hospital on the north coast of California as she went into labor. But the doctors were having none of it. Having a husband in the delivery room was out of the question. It was forbidden. In turn, *he* was having none of that—and promptly handcuffed himself to his wife. The police were called but could do little but watch as the woman gave birth while her husband was still chained to her.[1] Around the same time, another California man also protested his right to be at the birth of his child and was allowed into the delivery room only on the condition that he was strapped into a wheelchair that would be wheeled in by a nurse and plonked next to the delivery table.[2] Men weren't just regarded as a distracting spare part to be kept well away from the business of birth; those who wanted to be there were even seen as potentially deviant.[3] We were banished to the pub or other wombs of male sanctity. Every now and then, in the 1980s, an announcement would crackle over the tinny PA at the Manchester City soccer game: *Jim so-and-so in the North Stand, your wife has just given birth to a baby boy.* A big cheer, and then back to the beef extract drink that was oddly popular in the stands.

Good luck to the husband who nips off to watch sports these days when his wife goes into labor. While births were once a minority spectator sport for men—5 percent of fathers attended hospital births in the 1950s—today some 97 percent of husbands are present. And increasingly being hands-on. In the UK, the government encourages hospitals to have bigger birthing pools so fathers can wade right in too (duties include sieving out floating poos, I'm told).[4] My dad never touched a diaper in his life. Now men are bringing along fishing nets to births. We've come a long way.

The repurposing of tackle is the tip of a generational revolution in fatherhood. Men have never been so hands-on and emotionally present in bringing up kids. Could this be a golden era of fatherhood? On the other hand, presidents and popes warn that we're living through a "crisis of fatherhood."[5] We've never been good at doing things by halves.

In 1973, sperm counts were 99 million sperm per milliliter of semen; by 2011 that was down to 47 million per milliliter.[6] Some say between 1940 and 1990, the global quality decreased by half:[7] even our semen isn't impervious to the perils facing men today. Our depleted swimmers are under attack from every quarter: fried foods, pesticides, soy, phones, plastic bottles, vegetarianism, tight pants, yellow food dye, TV viewing, and breakfast muffins are just some of the seminal villains identified by the media recently. Our basic biological raison d'être put at risk by a Sara Lee cinnamon roll.[8] Never one to pass up the opportunity to adopt a new hypochondria, I've switched from soy milk to almond milk. Not just due to one sixty-year-old man developing breasts after drinking six pints of soya milk a day,[9] but because I would really like to be a dad. It's a pang I feel, with increasing intensity, when I see my niece and nephew and my friends' kids—well, the cuter ones at least. A male broodiness, that's almost on an emotional par with seeing the wet nose of a small gray Italian greyhound in the park.

It hardly takes an evolutionary biologist to sniff out where this urge to procreate must be coming from, in a man who really by now should be getting on with passing along his genetic material. Whether it's being a slave to the whim of one's DNA or not—and I know plenty of men and women who have no desire to disrupt their lives with kids, and good for them to forge their own paths—the feelings are real. As with religion, I don't unrealistically idealize parenthood. It looks like a relentless, exhausting, libido-killing, relationship-straining, time-sapping, identity-stealing mission that you muddle through without any manual. One that's easier if there's money to soften the edges and exponentially more stressful if you're struggling to make ends meet. All the while knowing that if you fail to nourish and sustain the relationship with your partner, while trying to pull off this parental balancing act, you're staring down the heartbreaking barrel of consigning your kids to divorce and weekend visits. And surely it's not too soon, without even having a partner yet, to preemptively worry about being one of the 10–20 percent of dads who seem to suffer from the little-understood *paternal* postnatal depression?[10]

Yet with all this trepidation duly noted, the little fellas are getting restless. I'm sure part of the reason why they're tired of swimming practice laps is that feeling—like seeing the people you grow up with virtually all get married—of being out of synch with where friends are at. Of wanting your kids to be able to play with theirs, not be babysat by them. Against that intangible background buzz of male competition, there's even a sense of being less of a man than those who have done their DNA homework on time.

Fatherhood seems to give aging a graceful framework too. That you can no longer name an act in the Top 40, last the full length of a football game, or be intuitively sure where skinny jeans fall on the line between hip and ridiculous is less of a cause for mourning when you've already completed the preening pretend-you've-still-got-it level and moved on to the next stage of the game. And that fatherhood level looks like it can be great fun, once more seeing the world through the prism of innocence and wonder, coupled with a massive dose of playful silliness. Friends with kids talk about falling in love all over again; how amazing it is to have that heart-filling sensation; what a realigning relief to relegate your own self-serving concerns below the real demands of someone who needs you; how it's a source of true long-term satisfaction and existential meaning whatever the short-term gripes and hassles.

I'm slightly grasping for generic platitudes to articulate a yearning for something that straddles the mundane and miraculous—and perhaps can only be accurately expressed once experienced. Once you've become that man who can't believe the same words his father said have mortifyingly reappeared in his own mouth. But from where I'm sitting in my loose-fitting undies, for all the ball ache of fatherhood, it looks like something to well and truly sacrifice the cinnamon rolls for.

* * *

In 1831, when fifteen-month-old baby Heman Wayland refused to stop crying and take a piece of bread being offered to him, his father Francis took this as a willful sign of refusal—and shut him in a room. For two days. He only let the baby out when the boy had not only eaten the bread but had also gladly opened his arms to his father. Francis, a Baptist minister and president of the Ivy League Brown University, outlined his doctrine of parenting thusly: "The Right of the parent is to command; the duty of the child is to obey."[11] And *he* was seen as liberal at the time, an educational modernizer and antislavery campaigner whose sons, including the incarcerated bread refusenik, later remembered with tenderness.[12]

Fathers have been austere, detached figures throughout history. In ancient Greece, men were expected not to show an active interest in their small children, with a commentary at the time castigating a master who dared to chew his baby's food—a task meant for the child's wet nurse—thus crossing a serious social boundary.[13] This was an admonishment dished up by a friend of Aristotle around 300 BC. In 1946, the child-rearing guru Dr. Spock advised fathers: "It's fine for him to do . . . things occasionally. He might make the formula on Sunday." So in the space of more than two millennia, fathers went from never touching baby food to maybe having a go once a week. But the intervening 2,000 years wasn't a straightforward linear progression to this giddy weekly bottle.

The closeness between fathers and their kids seems to have waxed and waned over time and across social classes. The distant disciplinarian father figure crops up in seventeenth-century England, where sons had to remain standing and daughters kneeling in a father's presence until otherwise instructed,[14] and in late nineteenth-century Pittsburgh where, in one family, the children were told to remain silent when the father was home.[15] Yet in the pre-Victorian years, fathers in novels and memoirs were being described with increased regularity as "tender."[16] Indeed, before industrialization dragged men off to factories, they'd often have been working at or near home—a daily presence in their children's lives and home for lunch.

The move toward modern fathering—and away from "Wait till your father gets home!"—is noticeable from the 1940s, when mothers began to assume the role of discipliner-in-chief and fathers took up the goofball play-around mantle. So intent were Dutch dads on taking this role seriously that "fathers' elbow" was named in honor of the dislocations caused during overzealous play.[17] But it's in the 1970s, following in the wake of those rather determined delivery room dads, that "new fathering" started to kick in.[18] Just as feminism in the 1970s, in its second wave, unleashed profound social changes that affect how women live today, was there a quiet yet powerful revolution in fathering also set in motion in that decade? One that means we now actually live in a golden era of fatherhood, quite unlike anything that's ever passed before?

SUPERDADS

We certainly spend more time with our kids than our fathers did with us, a majority of men report.[19] Not that that's hard to beat: research found working fathers in 1974 spent an average of five minutes a day dedicated to their children, which has now risen to thirty-five minutes of quality time (mothers clock up an hour).[20] Fathers have also rolled up their sleeves to bathe, feed, clothe, change diapers, help with homework, and ferry around children more than ever before. There are big variables across class and ethnicity—African American men in the US are much more likely than Hispanics to get involved with the bathing and diaper changing,[21] but fathers went from doing an average of 2.5 hours of childcare a week in 1965 to seven hours in 2011.[22] And the amount of male housework more than doubled—to ten hours a week—in the same period. (By comparison, combined childcare and housework for women comes in at thirty-two hours a week, down from forty-two hours in the midsixties, compared to seventeen hours for men.)

Beyond mere time metrics, there's been a seismic shift in the very essence of what it is to be a father. The hands-off, emotionally distant model looks increasingly like a Victorian relic. Children should now be seen and heard, with two-thirds of dads asking their children what they've been up to that day.[23] And once-stoic men are now racked with guilt: 46 percent of US fathers say they don't get to spend enough time with the children.[24] If anything, some fathers might be getting *too* involved—helicopter dads who have let their golf memberships slide to focus on pushing their kids toward greatness (kids who aren't going to be spending *their* childhoods being told to *just wait in the car*).

Sir Anthony Seldon, the recent headmaster at the British public school Wellington College, has seen this "mini-me" type. "They shout at the touchlines, they spend all their time at the school play videoing rather than watching the performance. This is a form of parental narcissism.

Rather than letting the child be what they want to be, they atrophy their child's sense of development and autonomy."

Tony Little, a former Eton College headmaster, has seen them too. "There has been a growth in some parents living their lives vicariously through their ambitions for their children. . . . For some, it feels like bereavement when something goes unexpectedly wrong; others are in denial."[25]

Well, that's what happens when you let infant mortality rates improve and allow parents to risk forming an emotional bond. None of that vicarious nonsense in the sixteenth century, when indifference reigned toward the children who survived infancy. The philosopher Montaigne, who lost five of his six daughters during infancy, wrote that he had learned to bear the loss of a child "not without regret, but without great sorrow."[26]

(ISH)

Before we high-five with our Playtex about how men have morphed into bionic superdads—soiled diaper in one hand, vacuum cleaner in the other, wishing if only *they* could lactate to share the cracked nipple burden—let's note the limits of this fathering revolution. We're not bashing the door down to have an equal share of child-rearing duties. In superliberal Sweden, the land where one party wanted to ban men in the council office from peeing standing up,[27] fathers only take 24 percent of the supergenerous parental leave.[28] Around a similar proportion, 21 percent, of the stay-at-home dads in the US (who have doubled since the late 1980s to around two million) say they're at home because they actually want to look after the kids; the vast majority are out of work, ill, disabled, or retired.[29] No matter how liberal the country, no matter that women now comprise 40 percent of the global workforce, women remain overwhelmingly more responsible for childcare and household duties.[30] Reasons for this beyond residual sexist piggery?

Financial? Men are still the biggest breadwinners, so it's in the family's best financial interests for them to go out to work (though this becomes a circular argument as women's careers are hit by, say, going part-time). If the man is working, then from a financial standpoint, it's worth the woman considering going back to work only if she'll earn more than the exorbitant cost of childcare. Of course, there are compelling nonfinancial reasons for women to want to return to work—independence, sanity, not wanting to be around young kids all day or risk seeing their career slip—which can make childcare costs particularly punitive.

I suspect the financial factor will hold less sway when today's youngsters come of working age. Those confident girls will no longer stand for this, probably overtaking male earnings anyway, with the future piecemeal way of employment meaning that men are more likely to have periods of being at home rather than disappearing into a nine-to-five vacuum for forty years.

Men are slackers? Knowing a woman will buckle first to sort out the kids or house. . . . Maybe this was true in those halcyon Don Draper days. In 1965, fathers did an average of 48.5 hours a week of combined paid work, house chores, and childcare—compared to a total of 51 hours for a woman. Today, Don would be choking on his scotch: fathers now do 1.5 hours a week more overall toil than mothers.[31] As one knackered father with two young kids said with a sigh: "The expectations on a modern dad with young kids are now overwhelming. You're expected to concurrently be the lead/sole breadwinner, find time to help with the morning drop-off, deliver a top performance at work, if possible get home to help with bath/bedtime, and potentially cook dinner. Then after a week of that, the weekend relaxation consists of 6:45 a.m. wake-up calls (if you're lucky), entertaining/playing with the kids before ferrying them (and in the early years accompanying them) to an array of children's soft-play parties. At about 8:30 p.m. on Sunday, your two-hour weekend break begins." He also says that when both parents are working, there's an unspoken "battle of hours" that hangs in the air each week over who has done more.

It's what people want? Dare it be said in this day and age, but maybe *some* couples are perfectly happy with the woman taking on the primary child-rearing role. Those maternal and paternal instincts, coupled with thousands of years of conditioning, are powerful drivers. Indeed, a Pew survey found "a strong majority"—62 percent—of working mothers in the United States would prefer to work part-time.[32] Tallying with this is the fact that in the US the number of stay-at-home moms has risen over the last fifteen years, and of these a quarter are now college-educated, women who perhaps could have chosen to work instead.[33] Stepping quickly away to male territory, polls suggest that only around a fifth of fathers want to be the ones raising the kids, while the vast majority still seek to be out there on traditional breadwinning duties, with all the accompanying identity and purpose that come from work, not to mention its outlet for competitiveness.[34] Maybe there's more than a hint of truth in the *New Yorker* cartoon in which a man stands before his boss and says, "My wife is about to have a baby, so I was wondering if you could make me work late for the next eighteen years or so."[35]

Frankly, babies don't do an awful lot for me—until they can get out a few words, puppies are still streets ahead. Research at Harvard Medical School suggests that while a woman tends to soothe a baby, a man is more likely to stimulate it. Men are also more likely to wait an extra second before rushing toward a toddler who has fallen over.[36] I'm sure there's no biological block, and we can pick up all the parental skills that are needed, but men, en masse, don't seem to be champing at the bit to be the main baby-rearers. Perhaps, as one mother of twins put it to me, paternal love can really come into its own as the children get older. To add to the list of pointless things to worry about while still being single, I'd also be concerned that if I stayed at home full-time with the kids, the sexual chemistry with my partner would be affected, no matter how sparkly I could get the taps.

Piss-poor paternity leave? If you really want to give men the chance to be more active in bringing up their kids—and bring more equal division to the labor—then let's get all Swedish. Not only did Swedish men see off attempts to curb *peeing erectus*, but they have also been granted up to 480 days of shared paternity leave, of which sixty days are reserved just for them. The result is that around 90 percent of Swedish dads take paternity leave, for an average of seven weeks, if not for their full entitlement.[37] If we're looking for reasons to ape our Scandi cousins, then researchers have found: it establishes an early bond that's more likely to endure (dads who take time off then tend to read to their kids more when they're toddlers); it can improve the child's performance as far down the line as secondary school, especially for daughters; it's good for the physical and mental well-being of the mother after birth; and it improves the mother's income. In Sweden, every month that fathers took paternity leave increased the mother's income by 6.7 percent when measured four years later.[38] Consultant psychiatrist Dr. Sebastian Kraemer has even found that the more parents are paid to care for their infants, the fewer baby boys, in particular, die (boys are born with greater vulnerability, he says).[39]

What's not to like? Surely, taking serious paternity leave is a no-brainer? Yet in the United States it's a no-*payer:* zero paid paternity leave is guaranteed (and, together with Papua New Guinea, the US is the only country to offer new moms no time off with pay).[40] Even Tunisia gives men a day's leave. In the UK, it's a paid fortnight, with some options now around splitting up to fifty-two weeks of shared parental leave. Only around half a dozen countries offer new fathers more than two weeks off. But no one comes close to touching those sensitive Vikings.

To take a step back from the stats, polls, paranoia about somehow implying that women deep down want to be at home, and limits to the sharing of burdens, the stand-out story is this fundamental reinvention of fatherhood in the West in the space of a generation or so. Today's modern dad role would be unrecognizable to nearly all our male ancestors. So can we herald this as a golden era?

I think what we can say is there's a golden *model* of fatherhood that's now on the table. A model that means a dad can be more involved in the lives and emotions of his children than ever before, if he wants to. Liberated from self-imposed and social shackles, fatherhood now comes with a healthy dose of freedom. Men are freer to stay at home with the kids, go part-time, dive into the birthing pool, run their own DaddyNatal classes, pick their children up from school without suspicious glances, express tenderness and emotion without fear that this somehow destroys all their authority, and have kids later in life. IVF, OVF, adoption, donated eggs, defrosted eggs—fatherhood comes in any number of permutations; straight and, hopefully with increasing ease, gay. (One freedom that is largely lacking, though, is the ability for a single man to have a child via a surrogate mother, the male equivalent of a partnerless woman using a sperm donor. Single men seeking to be biological dads seem to have to fly to California for the costly procedure in order to end up as sole guardians.)[41]

We are also strangely free of media-driven expectations of perfect fathers. If anything, the more common image is of the hapless, bumbling dad for whom the washing machine is a WMD-in-waiting. "To prove Huggies diapers and wipes can handle anything, we put them to the toughest test imaginable: Dads, alone with their babies, in one house, for five days."[42] What this 2012 Huggies ad *did* prove was that dads at least know how to operate a computer to petition against this demeaning guff, which then got pulled. But as long as there's a dearth of overcompetent and overattentive dads on our screens, as long as Homer Simpson lives on, we are less likely to feel like failures (and more likely to get excessive gratitude for a spot of housework). For years, the only program pumping the airwaves full of unrealistic expectations for how a father could somehow combine being a loving husband, doting dad, successful careerist, and great all-around guy who always kept a sense of humor was the *Cosby Show*, but I think we're in the clear now. (An Australian survey of the mass media found that only 12 percent of the reporting about men was favorable; most of the time we were portrayed as "villains, aggressors, perverts, and philanderers." And that was before the real Cosby show aired.[43])

So this model of fathering, with its unprecedented freedom to be the dad you want to be, is out there. But the model doesn't sit in a vacuum; it exists in the demanding, baffling world we live in. What affects how rewarding fatherhood actually can be are the realities and pressures that any good intentions might butt up against. Like being time poor. The unrelenting demands of today's workplace mean many fathers are missing out on the bath times and school plays they want to be at.[44] His situation is hardly typical, but chef Jamie Oliver and dad of four was far from alone when he told me, "Really, I'm a weekend dad, if the truth be told, which I think to be honest most busy modern-day men are." Men, women, superchefs— none of us can have it all. Interestingly, the country where men put in the most time helping out at home is France, where they are still on those hunter-gathering thirty-five-hour working weeks.[45]

Incidentally, here's Jamie's take on keeping the chemistry going when married with four kids: "As far as keeping the passion stuff alive, there's a natural sort of tempo to having a relationship, and it's not brilliant all the time. But it goes through lovely cycles if you trust and love each other . . . and I just think marriage is absolute comedy. To love someone so dearly but also despise them at the same time. We sometimes burst out in laughter 'cause we just can't stand each other at that moment. But we know each other so well, it's such a comfortable safe place."

Beyond time, money—and the widening gulf of inequality—will of course have an impact on fathering. Parenting will feel less like an ad for Disneyland if you're one of the 8.5 million families solely being fed by food stamps. Nor can being a dad be separated from the other pressures we've explored, like maintaining good mental health, meeting the challenge of monogamy, and keeping a healthy relationship afloat. Indeed, it's out of this wider brew of poverty, the negative effect of being unemployed or stuck in a dead-end job, a dearth of male role models, and failing relationships that the golden model loses its shine and that other modern phenomenon emerges: a crisis of fatherhood.

SUPERABSENT

Basically, an awful lot of kids are growing up without a father being around. When 15 million American children—one in three, and a majority of black kids—are growing up in homes without fathers,[46] with millions having zero contact at all,[47] when a million UK kids have no meaningful relationship with their fathers,[48] and there are "dad deserts" in places like the Liverpool ward that are 65 percent father-free, well, that's a crisis. If that needed confirming, Pope Benedict declared, "The crisis of fatherhood that we are experiencing today is a basic aspect of the crisis that threatens mankind as a whole."[49] The three US presidents up to Trump all weighed in too. If anyone was short of ammunition for the havoc being unleashed by absent fathers, children from dadless homes are more likely to excel at just about everything you don't want them to, from teen pregnancy to being adolescent murderers.[50] You could say that this crisis masks another crisis: poverty. As Kimmel notes, the higher the income bracket, the more likely the father is home.[51] Indeed, among US fathers who never completed high school, 40 percent live apart from their children, compared to only 7 percent of dads who graduated from college.[52]

Whether it's a symptom of poverty or not, the absence of dads is taking a terrible toll on kids and society. But among the myriad of individual reasons why fathers aren't present—men doing a runner, geographical separation, abusive histories (on either side), some men severing ties as a reaction to feeling rejected—there are plenty of dads screaming that it doesn't have to be this way. That they would do anything to see more of their kids. That fathers are being cut out by the courts.

In the kitchen of a west London café, a group of men is hovering around a stove with an intense concentration I've not seen since we were shown in tenth grade what happens when copper oxide reacts with magnesium. But there are no inorganic compounds holding their gaze, just all-purpose flour, milk, eggs, butter, and a pinch of salt. The dads are learning how to make a crêpe (and just how overpriced something is once you lob on a French accent). Brought together for practical support by the charity Dads House, they are all separated fathers who have a passion to not just spend every other Saturday afternoon staring at their kids over a box of soggy French fries in McDonald's. Like many a divorced dad, they're doing their best to step up. These aren't the feckless young men who shoot and leave. They're good guys trying to be better dads. Yet many of them have experienced periods that haunt them when they were denied access to their children. "I used to cry myself to sleep every night," says a gentle man in his early sixties who couldn't see his two young children for four years. Another guy, in his forties, was kept apart from his little boy. "It's a terrible feeling. It's such strange situation to be in—to have a heart full of love that you want to give to your child, but for some reason you're being blocked from doing that. It's not just the father that suffers but the child, ultimately." (Dads House also supports some of the 200,000 or so single fathers out there, some of whom are picking up the pieces in the more unusual instances of moms walking out on kids.)

Billy McGranaghan, the lithe Scotsman who founded Dads House, says that despite a change to UK law—so that courts will have to presume that the involvement of both parents after separation is in the child's best interest—"Things aren't getting better. If you have been refused access, it can take years to get access to your children. Dads have to be very careful how they contact their ex-partners. It's hard for dads, and it's heartbreaking as well." Men's rights campaigner Glen Poole also says studies showing that the courts don't discriminate against men are missing the point, given the meager level of access that many are winning. "Our expectation of the role a separated father should play in his children's lives is so low that when half of dads who win 'access' to their kids can't even sleep under the same roof as their offspring, academics declare this to be an overwhelming success."[53]

It's complex, messy, emotional stuff, but it seems the momentum is at last moving in a dad-friendly coparenting direction. Legislatures in more than twenty states considered bills in 2017 that would encourage shared parenting or make it a legal presumption—even when parents disagree. In superprogressive Sweden, a third of children whose parents aren't together are now being brought up in "shared residency," dividing their week between living with Mom and Dad. However, coparenting isn't a panacea and is not always in a child's best interests, and Swedish research has found it's important to give the child a voice in any shared arrangements. As one kid said, "Mom and Dad decide, but I tell them if it's no good."[54]

I have a strange litmus test for being the sort of father I'd want to be. I imagine my mythical child, when they are grown up, lying on a therapist's couch. The shrink is asking them what I was like as a parent. If all they've got to whine about is the run-of-the-mill screwups, embarrassments, and arguments, then that's a job well done. If they can't pinpoint any actual fuckuppery, I'll be happy.

When envisaging what kind of father you aspire to be, it's only natural to reflect on your own upbringing. What from your father would you want to emulate, and what would be best left in a parenting box in the attic? I'd be in no rush to unpack the impulse to marry someone I'd only met six weeks earlier, nor the experiment with how long a teenager can survive when only fed broken cookies. For all my dad's idiosyncrasies—and customer service experiences that would make Larry David blush—there are core traits I deeply cherish.

Resilience: Only as an adult can I now truly appreciate what it must have been like to lose your wife and shortly afterward go through a divorce, all the while trying to run your own business and bring up two boys. But he really kept his shit together.

Supportiveness: Full marks for the love, encouragement, and support.

Creativity: The photographs of Sefton Samuels are truly stunning.

Maverickness: From taking up yoga in the 1950s to turning up to his wedding with his best man on a tandem, both wearing top hats, he's been his own man.

Empathy: Generous even when there wasn't much of a pot to piss in and really sticking by people who have had a hard time. These latter two traits combined recently when, so frustrated with the plight of Kris Maharaj still being in jail in Florida, he wrote to President Obama offering to swap places with Kris in prison.

Even as an allegedly emotionally articulate male, I can still only seem to express the love I have for my father in cursory list form. I blame the parents.

OH BOY

One crisis—fatherhood—isn't enough for males these days. Like a man-size box of Kleenex, or a Gillette razor crying out for yet another blade, a man can always squeeze in a bit more.

If the lucky one of your 300 million or so stragglers that made it up the ampulla to fertilize an egg was carrying the Y chromosome, then congratulations, you've contributed to this other crisis. You've formed a boy.

This crisis among boys vexes governments from Australia to (heaven forbid) Sweden. Book titles refer to *Hear Our Cry* and *Saving Our Sons.* A

Newsweek cover declaimed "The Boy Crisis," while the *Atlantic* referred to "The War Against Boys."[55] There's no shortage of ammunition to show the plight of young males. Although plenty of perfectly functional and nice young men are being brought up, boys are:

- Lagging behind in reading in every state at elementary, middle, and high school levels[56] and an average of a year behind in reading alone in all sixty-four countries measured by the OECD.
- Around a third less likely to go to college.
- Three times more likely to be expelled from high school.
- Six times more likely to be diagnosed with ADD.
- Four times more likely to be diagnosed as "emotionally disturbed" or attempt suicide.
- Fifteen times more likely to be the victim of a violent crime.[57]
- Getting heavier: a third of boys are either overweight or obese.[58]

Who'd want to bring up one of these chubby bundles of statistical crises, instead of a nice conscientious girl who'll do all her reading and then get a better degree to support you in old age? Perhaps that's why one fertility clinic in the US reports that eight in ten of the British couples who have a gender choice there (which is not available back home) choose to have a girl.[59] And why girls are consistently preferred to boys by adoptive parents in the United States.[60] Boys have been prized throughout history at the brutal expense of baby girls—which still persists in parts of China and India—but will modern designer parenting one day induce a boy shortage? Pandas holding telethons for endangered human boys? (While working-class white boys become ever more detached from educational achievement and the chance to make it in the modern economy, the College Board advocacy center chillingly noted: nearly half of young men of color ages fifteen to twenty-four who graduate from high school will end up unemployed, incarcerated, or dead.[61])

This boy crisis feels like a sign of our modern times, but we've had hints of this before. In 1900, girls were preferred as adoptees.[62] Indeed, the 1916 annual report of the Spence-Chapin adoption service in New York states, "We now have on file sixty-one applications, of which six are for boys, fourteen for either sex and forty-one for girls. Why do so many people prefer girls! The majority seem to feel that a girl is easier to understand and to rear, and they are afraid of a boy."[63] It was around this time that fears about the physical and moral fiber of boys—especially the corrupting, feminizing impact of schools staffed by women—threw up the Scouts, YMCA, and the whole muscular Christian notion that standing on a sodden rugby field could save a British lad's soul (and the Empire). The Indiana senator Albert Jeremiah Beveridge decried in 1906 the whole idea of boys passively learning in classrooms, urging them to "avoid books and in fact avoid all artificial learning, for the forefathers put America on the right path by learning completely from natural experience."[64]

He may have been overcooking it by suggesting that boys dispense with books, but was the senator onto something? If he were around today, he'd find that not only have his worst fears of young men being failed by the education system been realized and then some, but also that many people have come around to his way of thinking and oppose cramming boys into passive classrooms all day, arguing that boys, whether posh or poor, have different needs from girls. As the former Wellington College head puts it, "It's all to do with their brains and bodies and chemicals."[65]

Some indeed home in on the physiological. Girls, supposedly, hear better than boys, who therefore should be seated near the front of the class. The optimal temperature for boys to learn in is 69°F (20.5°C), whereas for girls it is 75°F (24°C).[66] In addition, males simply need to move about more.

"Boys do have higher activity levels, and it's because their brains were washed in androgens (male sex hormones) before they were born," notes psychologist Dr. Michael Thompson, an expert on the development of boys. "By the time school starts, three-quarters of the boys in class are more physically active, more impulsive, and, let's face it, more developmentally immature than girls of the same age. That's a real biological difference."[67]

If there is this difference, put simply, should we be teaching boys differently? Studies support the idea of harnessing boys' competitive spirit and getting them moving more in lessons.[68] But what specifically can be done to avert whole swathes of disengaged boys joining the swelling ranks of depressed, angry men who haven't got the skills to make it in the modern economy (hopefully they'll avoid joining the United State Postal Service at a time of restructuring)? Dr. Thompson, who says so many boys find school "irrelevant and inauthentic," suggests promoting "meaningful responsibility" by:

- Giving boys, from early on, responsibility for taking care of animals, such as chickens or rabbits that need daily care.
- From a very young age, putting boys in charge of younger children—reading to them, running games, coaching sports, and being trained as lifeguards, referees, and umpires.
- Allowing boys in the last two years of high school the option of swapping some classroom lessons for training in the workplace, responding to the "universal boy need to be useful, to do something that is actually respected in the world." Some German high schools send kids off to work in a Mercedes plant in the afternoon; working alongside adults in an actual workplace is "what many boys need."

He also recommends outdoor and wilderness expeditions. Maybe we could address our failure to mark boys' transition to manhood by integrating into school life a modern-day rites of passage program; the Australian Rite Journey, for example, takes pupils on a seven-stage mental and physical challenge across the year, culminating in a solo wilderness experience.[69]

For our utopian boy-friendly education, other gurus have suggested:

- More freedom at times to roam, to play, to fight (in controlled contexts, such as martial arts). And giving boys an awareness of how the human mind and emotions work (Marek Kazmierski, a former governor at Feltham Young Offenders Institution).
- Support teacher training in how boys' and girls' brains learn differently, which leads to better behavior and results for both (Michael Gurian, author of *The Minds of Boys*).
- Have a stream of men come into school and share their stories—men who look like them, who they can relate to, who show there's more than one way to be masculine other than doing drugs or ending up in prison. Bring in successful guys, gay guys, guys who have tackled mental illness. Allow boys to ask, "Am I choosing my masculinity or is it choosing me?" (Brandon Hay, Black Daddies Club, Toronto).

That's some school taking shape.

CHIP OFF THE OLD BLOCK

The "boy crisis" in the classroom and beyond seems like a junior version of the wider pressures affecting men today; the Happy Meal waiting to be precociously supersized. The man/boy parallels are striking.

- Men trapped at their desks in offices; boys stuck on their bums all day in class. Both entirely out of touch with their biological design.
- Men suppressing maverick or overly competitive instincts to advance in the modern workplace; boys who are rough around the edges being marked down in the modern classroom. There's evidence that boisterous boys receive lower grades from their teachers than testing would have predicted, with a grade "bonus" awarded to those boys who behave like the nice girls in class.[70] And boys who play how boys have always played—making grenade noises or fashioning a gun out of a saccharine breakfast snack—might not even get to stay in the classroom at all.
- Men in societies sanitized from risk driven to extreme and sometimes self-destructive lengths to get the sensation-seeking fixes that used to be a natural part of hunter-gathering life; boys being cocooned from risk and nature. Not being allowed to roam outside, play rough, or climb trees, boys spend so little time outdoors that half can't tell the difference between a bee and a wasp.[71]

Take the humble tree. An indispensable vantage point for spying on baddies for the *Famous Five*. "[Dick] debated where to hide and then made a quick decision," writes Enid Blyton in the 1950 classic *Five Fall into Adventure*. "I'll climb a tree. . . . I could perhaps catch a glimpse of what the man's like who comes to collect the parcel. Then I'll shin quietly down the tree and stalk him."[72] If Enid Blyton had been setting this in the West Midlands today, Dick and his friends would have been arrested, had their shoes removed, photos taken, and DNA samples fed into the police system. Yes, that really happened to three eleven- and twelve-year-olds caught

red-handed building a den in a cherry tree (which was suffering branch damage from the ordeal).[73] When not being the
scene of major crime incidents, trees are places where children
develop their own "risk thermostats." By experiencing that it's
harder to climb down than up, they're learning how to judge
risk themselves.[74] Half of kids in England have been stopped
from climbing trees, the National Children's Bureau found.[75]
Another reason to make us hug the nearest deciduous: expo-
sure to nature reduced symptoms in children with attention
deficit hyperactivity disorder (ADHD)—that particularly
boy-prone disorder—threefold compared with staying
indoors, a study found.[76] If I have a boy, he's bloody well living in a tree house.

- Men's minds being filled with entirely unrealistic expectations
for what they should be achieving in life, contributing to serious mental health issues; boys failing to cope with the pressures they're under. We can see this from boys as young as two
to eight years old being more likely than girls to have a mental,
behavioral, or developmental disorder and from studies showing that eating disorders are growing twice as fast among boys
as girls, especially boys aged between ten and fourteen (though
such disorders are still ten times more common in girls, who
are also experiencing truly torrid emotional pressures).[77]

  The head teacher of the top-rated Royal Grammar School
  in Newcastle says academic pressures are driving boys to
  anorexia. "It tears me up to see bright, attractive, talented
  youngsters who cannot take joy in their achievements because
  of their anxiety. I would like to shout at them, 'Do you not
  realize how good you are?'"[78]

- Men no longer feeling part of a tribe struggling to find that
sense of belonging and identity elsewhere, even being drawn

to conflict and extreme ideologies; boys falling under the spell of gangs or at least fitting in by going along with the male mentality that "it's not cool for them to perform, it's not cool to be smart," in the words of a Bronx head teacher.[79] "There are different pressures on boys. . . . Unfortunately, there's a tendency where they try to live up to certain expectations in terms of [bad] behavior."

If these are tough times to be a boy, it's not least because these are strange days. For most of the time that young men have been lolling around this planet, their main focus would have been perfecting the arts of survival and hunting, learning how to spear a bison or wild cattle. Now, in those unchanged cave-boy bodies, whose eyes are still better at viewing distant objects than the female's,[80] they can't climb a tree or tell a bee from a wasp. Their boisterous fearlessness, inculcated through many an agonizing ritual initiation, was once lauded by women. Celtic warriors used to be greeted back from battle by women baring their breasts[81]; now women teachers mark down boys for being too rowdy. Once, boys would have grown up in tight bands alongside role-model fathers and guiding elders. Now, vast numbers barely have contact with their fathers, and elders and their wisdom have been banished out of sight to residential care homes. Young heads that used to have a (perhaps entitled) sense of solid roles and secure futures ahead are wavering under the pressures of test-driven academia, social media judgment on their popularity and body image, toxic porn-fueled sexual expectation, a near-religious exaltation of fame, and a looming job market in which many will be ill-equipped to thrive.

When boys are faced with such a dizzying array of challenges that cut to the heart of modern masculinity, there are clearly limits to what even the most enlightened school or well-meaning parent can achieve. Indeed, has there ever been a time when fathers and mothers have had so little control over the influences that sway their device-savvy children? Outside school and whatever tidbits my friends might have picked up, my main pipeline of information was the TV, which my dad had the power to control and ultimately switch off (as happened the instant the first televised boob I ever saw popped out on screen).

How analogue.

To make a real impact on the plight of boys, schools and parents could do with some heavy-lifting from the rest of society: throwing the onus on social media, advertising agencies, and food companies to ensure that whatever is being pumped into children's heads and bodies is more nourishing than destructive; providing serious mentoring for boys who are growing up without a father figure; and giving the elderly more of a presence in kids' lives, such as placing childcare and nurseries in retirement homes.

Crucially, giving dads every chance to be the best they can be in a time when they've never had such potential to be so close to their kids: to allow long paternity breaks for those who want it, to not deny dads access unless there's a truly compelling reason, to be creative with custody, and to roll out fatherhood classes for those who lack confidence or skills. Obama (whose dad was largely absent after he was two) dropped half a billion dollars into funding hundreds of fathering classes, saying, "What makes you a man is not the ability to have a child, it's the courage to raise one."[82]

And just to remember that, from the day they are born and bite harder on the mother's nipple, boys are different.[83]

13
CONCLUSION: RECLAIM THE SPEAR

Mohamed Bouazizi's day started as usual. The twenty-six-year-old woke early in the tiny three-bedroom house he shared with his mother, uncle, and five brothers and sisters, went to load his wooden cart with fruit from the market, then pushed it a mile to his habitual spot on a street in the town of Sidi Bouzid in central Tunisia. For his day's labors, he'd expect to earn the usual five or so dollars, with which he'd somehow have to support all eight of them and keep his sisters in school. His dreams were modest: to own a van to transport the fruit in. Maybe that morning his mind had strayed to his soccer team, Esperance Sportive, or hopes of one day getting married. Or perhaps to the lack of other options to earn a living in a town where even the academics worked the land, where legions of young men were unemployed, and where getting a job in the local tomato paste factory required connections.

Just after 11 a.m., he was confronted with the bane of his life, the officialdom that routinely got in the way of his meager five dollars a day. Because no one would grant him a vending permit, sometimes he'd be hit with a steep bribe or arbitrarily have his stall shut down. That morning, as he sold his tangerines, apples, and pears, a female municipal officer, with a reputation for being strict, approached Mohamed to confiscate his goods and electric scales. Other vendors say that as he tried to wrestle his apples back, the female inspector slapped Mohamed across the face.

A public slap in the face, by a woman, in a deeply proud and patriarchal society. (I'll see your being shouted at by a woman boss in the office and raise that with a slap and loss of income.)

Enraged, Mohamed walked a few blocks to the municipal office to demand his property back—and was turned away. He asked to see the governor, but was again turned away. At lunchtime, he then took his wooden cart to the street in front of the governor's office, poured a bottle of paint thinner over his head, and set himself on fire. An act of self-immolation that claimed his life and sparked the Arab Spring. Regimes toppled in Tunisia, Egypt, Libya, and Yemen; ripples spread to Bahrain, Saudi Arabia, and Mali; and the Syrian civil war broke out, creating the world's worst refugee crisis since the Second World War and putting ISIS on the map. Mohamed, the everyman martyr, a symbol of the oppression borne by so many, lit one heck of a fuse of discontent. The assault by the female official became legend, even if it was only that (as she claims).

Just as the assassination of Archduke Franz Ferdinand set in motion the outbreak of the First World War, was the Arab Spring—and its profound global repercussions that are still playing out across Syria and Yemen—triggered by the humiliating slap across a man's face?[1]

Never underestimate the male capacity for self-destruction in the face of thwarted attempts to be a breadwinner, especially when humiliation or shame is thrown into the mix. Mohamed's actions were extreme by any standards but not entirely without context: in the two years up to his death, 10,000 recession-related suicides had taken place across the United States and Europe. These were men in the US, UK, Germany, etc., from radically different backgrounds than a Tunisian fruit vendor, but who were all driven to the darkest despair by their work situations, perhaps infused with an accompanying sense that they had failed as men.

It all fits into a wider setting.

I posed the question at the beginning of this book of whether masculinity was like a Whac-A-Mole game, resiliently popping up elsewhere whenever it's suppressed. I am now more convinced of this than ever. Masculinity is a powerful force, an energy that courses through men (at differing levels according to individuals and their ages). An energy that has its roots in both our biological wiring—with our brains washed in androgens before we've even been born—and countless generations of conditioning and competing.

When harnessed and given purpose, it can be a tremendous force for action and positivity, driving males to be overrepresented among the highest achievers: running countries and companies, making scientific and tech breakthroughs. But without an outlet or direction, that same force can turn in on itself or become outwardly destructive, leading to violence and mental health problems as well as the male overrepresentation in prisons. "More Nobels and dumbbells—and that is the story of males," as the philosopher Dr. Cronin said.

This vital force, as we've seen, has a habit of popping up all over the place when unable to vent. Young men, with no rite to mark the passage to manhood, losing their virginities ever younger, and enduring extreme gang and frat initiations (hazing killed at least ten members of the Sigma Alpha Epsilon fraternity in the last decade).[2] Schoolboys who aren't given the chance to burn off energy, learn actively, or be boisterous, acting up, falling behind, and dropping out, with attention spans shot to pieces. The yearning for risk-taking being sated by hammering cars, dangling off cliffs, and having affairs. Men cooped up in offices feeling alive again only once they're taking punches. The craving to belong, to be part of a tribe, driving young men to join gangs and ISIS, old men to lapse into untreated depression when cast aside from the clan in a residential care home, and corporate men to sing the KPMG anthem.

Thwarted masculinity that sees some men pay $3,000 to learn how to gorge on compensatory sex and others to quite literally feel the need to flaunt their manliness in the cascade of cockshots abounding on Tinder. Libidos and urges grappling with monogamy but all too often ending in breakup. Self-destructive self-medication through drugs, alcohol, porn, overwork, and an unknown level of eating disorders. Eruptions of anger in mass shootings—and the rage against the concocted enemies comprising women, minorities, and immigrants. Trump. The Wall. Brexit. Guns.

But if ever proof were needed of this Whac-A-Mole masculinity, it came during an interview with a plastic surgeon on Harley Street in London. It happened to be a particularly intrusive interview about men and plastic surgery, and the producer thought it would make great radio for me to have a full examination during the chat. So while I dropped my pants and the doctor had a good old look, he casually made reference to something extraordinary. "Interestingly, after the 2008 financial crisis, the number of penile augmentations skyrocketed because men felt very, very insecure."

* * *

Masculinity is a primal, irrepressible force, then, that can drive men to the presidency, prison, and even penoplasty. What to do with this knowledge?

Well, if the men who comprise 98 percent of self-made billionaires and 95 percent of the Fortune 500 CEOs,[3] or who scooped all the 2015 Nobel prizes bar literature (and a quarter of the peace accolade), were representative of how this male spirit is being deployed, then we wouldn't have to do an awful lot. We'd congratulate ourselves on how our timeless competitive and "doing" instincts can be harnessed for greatness (while putting fingers in our ears if anyone mentioned "glass ceilings"). But in this era of extreme inequalities, the men at the top—who populate the 0.1 percent, though not without their own neuroses—are almost a different species of male than the guys working their asses off to make ends meet or pull off a half-decent quality of life. If anything, it's the dumbbell variant of masculinity that seems to be getting a good stretch these days.

For many men, the stool is a bit wobbly.

And not surprisingly. Our lives—and what fills our heads—would be unrecognizable to just about every one of our male ancestors. In the last generation or two alone, virtually every aspect of life has undergone radical change—our work, relationships, sex, fathering, faith, free time, connection to women, and what we feel we *should* be doing.

It's not all woe-is-man, harking back to some nonexistent halcyon era of pipe-and-slippers male contentment. If freedom is the badge of men's desires, then in some ways we are less restricted than ever in becoming the type of man we want to be. The male menu now includes hands-on, loving, superrewarding fathering; stay-at-home dads; rich relationships rooted in being equal partners; gay marriage and greater sexual liberty; being able to emotionally express how you feel beyond just grunting. And less chance than ever of being sent off to war.

Yet freedom feels in short supply for the man commuting to spend his days as a 360-degree-appraised cog in a hermetically sealed office, who barely has time to see his family or friends; for the lad who is the third generation of unemployed males in his family, for whom social mobility is a traffic jam that's not budging; for the boys who can't climb trees; and for the more than 800,000 black men locked up in a US jail cell today.[4] Not to mention all those of us who are hostage to the *shoulds* clamoring away in our heads.

Freer, yet in some ways more trapped than many a time before. The strange, not always refreshing taste, of Man Zero.

GOOD-FOR-SOMETHING

Back to the idea of ourselves as wobbly stools—and what can make us more robust, especially now that the work leg is looking shakier than ever and the buffeting of expectations shows no sign of dying down. As well as the regular supports—like relationships, family, friends, physical and mental health, wealth, community, Western and Eastern belief systems—we should add another leg: masculinity. Or, more specifically, "Good Masculinity."

We rarely stop to think about masculinity, other than with the prefix "toxic" or in relation to #MeToo: paradoxically it's ubiquitous yet invisible. Why fret about male traits when men, as a cohort, are still dominant? Having been a prized asset throughout time—a quality to herald when having to raise armies to fight wars or go colonizing—traditional, muscular masculinity has, if anything, taken on the whiff of outdated irrelevance; an obstacle to progress best left in the 1970s. The mutton-chopped, bottom-pinching relative who'd be the last person you'd call for advice on how to get ahead in today's world.

But what we've lost sight of is the innate, enduring power of masculinity, and how it can be channeled as a force for good. Think of the guys with crippling anxiety who can face the world again thanks to putting on boxing gloves. Or how violent crime and reoffending rates have been slashed among the wayward Chicago kids who took up after-school sports and the young British men who headed into the wilderness with mentors. Or the research that suggests that men who meet their buddies socially twice a week are healthier and recover more quickly from illness.[5] Or how reversing the direction of unemployment rates among young men has helped stabilize peace in Northern Ireland.

A positive channeling of this force is good not just for us, but those around us. A man grounded in who he is, where restlessness, anger, and frustrations are quelled, will be a better husband/partner/father. Conversely, the self-destructive man leaves those closest to him—and society as a whole—to pick up the pieces. Part of the kindness and generosity that experts suggest underpin a good relationship should be an encouragement for a man to be able to vent his good masculinity. Let men be men. If it helps, just occasionally visualize that beneath the suit, moisturized skin, and love handles lies the physiology of an unreconstructed wooly-mammoth killer (though odds are, he'd have returned with near-miss stories and be reliant on the fruit and grubs that the women had more likely foraged). Likewise, men should be generous in supporting whatever makes their partners most robust, even if that puts us out of our comfort zones, and no matter how similar our desires are in these convergent days.

Put simply, we need to give our *good masculinity* a proper workout. What was once naturally kept in shape through our lifestyles has grown flabby in today's way of living. This isn't a call for Flintstones regression therapy; salvation doesn't lie in a return to the cave. But as we go about our modern lives, it's to remember where we've come from, how we've been living and conditioned over the last 200,000 years, and the evolutionary design of the bodies we're walking around in. It's absurd not to factor this into our lives, but it is just *a* factor. One leg of the stool—albeit one that complements the others—alongside all the good stuff we've picked up since leaving the cave.

Nor does masculinity equal machismo or subjugating others. This isn't calling for life to be one long bachelor party. There are smart, modern, enlightened ways to tap into this drive. A yearning to be part of a tribe, for example, could be expressed by taking a decent wedge of paternity leave or spending time with elders. There isn't a single prescription; it's about individuals finding whatever works for them to channel this force. I know mine will be very different, and somewhat lower altitude, than my brother's.

You can feel it in yourself when you're in flow with that good masculinity, that sense of being alive and alert, infused with purpose. And you can see it in others—there's a certain infectious energy in a man comfortable in his own skin. Likewise, you can spot in many an office or job center the listless pallor of men out of kilter with their drive. Interestingly, some of the most passion-sapped men I've seen have been maximum security prison guards in the US, whose very job is to ensure other men are deprived of their freedom.

Of late, my man energy would certainly qualify for the correctional facility gig. It's been a chastening personal experience to explore in depth what makes a man robust; my stool feels more like a pogo stick. *Could do better* would be the verdict on just about every front (and the abnormally isolating nature of writing has been a challenge). I'd wager that the physiological signs of good masculinity don't extend to having near-constant pins and needles down the left arm from being hunched over a computer like a winded monkey, or a clicky right thumb from over-Tindering during writing breaks (early-onset arthritis from swiping?). Nor, the other day, did it feel like the whole settling-down mission was being taken seriously as I spent the evening trying to tease out whether the hot date was in fact too fascist to pull: wanting to build a fence to keep Muslims out of Europe didn't bode well. Why do I keep attracting fascists? Are they trying to round me up?

I bet motivational guru Tony Robbins doesn't reach the end of his books and think, *Shit, I've got an awful lot to change in life* (unless he really hadn't the foggiest beforehand that *"The only limit to your impact is your imagination and commitment"*—that'll be $480 million, please). And he'd probably come up with a really useful checklist too to round things off with. (Um, I actually spent time recently filming with and interviewing Tony Robbins and am pleased to report that he is an inspiring and self-deprecating chap. Oops.)

AND STRETCH

We go through our days counting the calories we eat. The steps we take. If we've had our five fruit and veg a day. But we don't stop to consider whether we've done enough to sate our masculinity—this fundamental, powerful force we barely acknowledge yet which seems to have such profound consequences depending on how it's channeled. These are baffling times to be a man; we live in a world rich in potential but laden too with pitfalls that can send men spiraling. It can traverse both great laughs and serious struggles. For all our outward dominance—and some guys are doing very nicely indeed—a lot of individual men are having a tough time, and many more are getting along but could be having a better time. And couldn't we all benefit from being a bit more grounded or having more moments when we feel alive?

Governments, companies, schools, and the media can all do more to improve the lives of boys and men: tackling the roots of why so many end up in jail, flunk out of school, and are in dire states of mental health; ensuring an economic future and social mobility regardless of class or race; obliterating the open-plan office; helping fathers be as present as they want to be and skilled for the job; bringing older people back into our lives; stopping portraying us as two-dimensional oafs and pumping our heads full of silly expectations about relationships, romance, and success.

As a society, we need to make masculinity—the *right* form of masculinity—fashionable again. It was championed when there were wars to fight; now it can be nurtured and deployed for the serious domestic struggles we're facing.

But we can also take individual responsibility in making ourselves stronger and happier—the best versions of ourselves. Alongside whatever else we know makes us robust and content, we can actively cultivate our own good masculinity. To see this as a vital force to nourish. A muscle that needs exercising.

While there are myriad ways and forms for different men to channel this force, I'd say there are underlying core strands. So each week, as well as counting what you've eaten or how much exercise you've done, maybe monitor how much good masculinity has been flexed. To summon the inner caveman: how many Spears you've earned.

WEEKLY SPEARS (1 SPEAR FOR EACH TASK)

Be productive:
- ⚡ Master/improve a skill (that has nothing to do with work but still make you feel like you're growing).
- ⚡ Be absorbed in a task/hobby that builds, makes, or fixes something.

Be in the body/unleash positive aggression:
- ⚡ Play sports.
- ⚡ Learn a martial art.
- ⚡ Do yoga or meditation.
- ⚡ Take part in a controlled-risk activity.

Be reminded of a man's place in the world:
- ⚡ Engage with nature or head into the wilderness (and look up).
- ⚡ Look after an animal.

Be with your pack:
- ⚡ Socialize with a male friend.
- ⚡ Socialize with four-plus male friends at once, especially over a joint activity.

Be with your minitribe:
- ⚡ Spend quality time with children/young relatives. Make elders feel part of the family.
- ⚡ Unplug and eat together.

Be part of a bigger tribe/sense of belonging:
  ⚡ Attend a communal gathering/crowd of like-minded people (that's not work-related).
  ⚡ Sing at that gathering.
  ⚡ Do something for a cause you believe in. Mentor or teach someone.

BONUS SPEARS

⚡ Express emotion, admit to fears/vulnerability, or ask for help.
⚡ Call out hatred.
⚡ Have sex with a woman/partner who feels free and fulfilled in life.
⚡ Use the postcome clarity window to be honest about your own sexual needs.
⚡ Actually approach a girl you like the look of when sober (if single).

Penalty Spears (-1 Spear each)
  ⚡ Watch any porn that features an egg.
  ⚡ Eat Corn Flakes.
  ⚡ Eat Corn Flakes with soy milk.
  ⚡ Cry at work.

Is six Spears a week too much to ask?

My great-grandfather saved his whole family by shipping them to England, away from the murderous riots that were erupting in the old Russian Empire. My grandfather served in the British Army during the First World War. My father survived the blitzes of the Second World War and faced down some heavy-duty adversities. When the men before us have fought life-and-death battle—had medals pinned to their chests—how are we to prove ourselves? How can we, as all men crave, be called *heroes*?

War has been the age-old shortcut to heroism, to achieve that feeling of total meaning. Thankfully, most of us aren't ever going to see battle. But there are other routes to being a hero; indeed, the need to equate heroism with conflict, in order to raise armies and support war efforts, may have thrown us off the scent for what good masculinity can actually look like. We might not be facing direct existential threats on the scale of our fore-fathers, but we have some serious fights on our hands, from big social injustices to merely trying to carve out our own fair share of contentment. And we can only beat what's in front of us. Heroism can be found close to home. In the everyday acts of being a father, partner, friend, or worker that can make a difference to those around us, and maybe even leave the world a slightly better place. No one is going to pin a medal on *our* chests. The rewards are going to come from a grateful smile, an energizing moment of being alive—and feeling true to the men we are.

ACKNOWLEDGMENTS

I am deeply grateful to a lot of women, and a few men.

For the initial vision and guidance this side of the Pond: Rowan Lawton, Rory Scarfe, Ben Dunn, Kate Raybould, Selina Walker, and Pippa Wright.

To Cal Barksdale—and everyone at Skyhorse Publishing—for masterfully and lovingly sailing this opus across the Atlantic. To Shannon Hassan for her invaluable work.

For providing invaluable wisdom and encouragement, thanks to Noreena Hertz, Gloria Abramoff, Jemima Khan, and Janet Lee. For doing years of top-notch academic cogitation around masculinity that I could then help myself to, I salute the genius of Michael Kimmel and Tony Rotundo.

To my father Sefton, brother Mark, current maternal figure Ann, and all my mates and family: your belief and love is the greatest leg a stool could ever hope for. To the terrible dates: sorry, but thanks for the stories.

And my everlasting gratitude to the *mohel* for keeping a steady hand during my first brush with masculinity.

NOTES

1. INTRODUCTION: WHO STOLE MY SPEAR?

1. http://www.greatfallstribune.com/story/news/local/2014/11/02
   /abarr-proposes-inclusive-kkk-chapter-mt/18397651/.
2. http://apps.who.int/iris/bitstream/10665/77428/1/WHO_RHR
   _12.41_eng.pdf.
3. https://nationalwomenshistoryalliance.org/resources/womens
   -rights-movement/detailed-timeline/.
4. *Women in Public Life: Gender, Law and Policy in the Middle East and North Africa* (OECD Publishing, 2014).
5. http://www.thenational.ae/uae/courts/court-rules-on-domestic
   -discipline.
6. Kimmel, Michael S., *The History of Men: Essays on the History of American and British Masculinities* (Albany: SUNY Press, 2005).
7. https://www.cdc.gov/healthequity/lcod/men/2015/all-males/index
   .htm.
8. Starr, Sonja B., "Estimating Gender Disparities in Federal Criminal Cases," University of Michigan Law and Economics Research Paper (August 29, 2012), no. 12-018.

9. Ruspini, Elisabetta, et al., eds., *Men and Masculinities around the World* (New York: Palgrave Macmillan, 2011), 161.

10. http://www.theatlantic.com/sexes/archive/2013/05/when-men-experience-sexism/276355/.

11. http://www.ncbi.nlm.nih.gov/pmc/articles/PMC3018605/.

12. https://www.hudexchange.info/resources/documents/2016-AHAR-Part-1.pdf.

13. https://www.cdc.gov/violenceprevention/nisvs/2015NISVSdatabrief.html.

14. http://www.theguardian.com/lifeandstyle/2008/aug/03/gender.healthandwellbeing.

15. http://www.telegraph.co.uk/news/health/news/10978836/Number-of-women-travelling-to-America-to-choose-sex-of-child-rises-20.html.

16. http://timesofindia.indiatimes.com/city/nagpur/Man-jailed-for-one-year-in-adultery-case/articleshow/18422997.cms.

2. BECOMING A MAN
(IN THE SAFEWAY PARKING LOT)

1. http://www.artofmanliness.com/2010/02/21/male-rites-of-passage-from-around-the-world/ and http://www.orijinculture.com/community/masculinisation-dehumanization-sambia-tribe-papua-guinea/.

2. Neusner, Jacob, ed., *World Religions in America: An Introduction*, 4th ed. (Louisville, KY: Westminster John Knox Press, 2009), 16.

3. Bly, Robert, *Iron John: A Book About Men* (London: Rider, 1990), 14.

4. Thanks to the thoughts of Professor Astrid Blystad at the University of Bergen.

5. Arnold, John and Sean Brady, eds., *What Is Masculinity?: Historical Dynamics from Antiquity to the Contemporary World* (New York: Palgrave Macmillan, 2011), 251.

6. Thamuku, Masego and Marguerite Daniel, "The Use of Rites of Passage in Strengthening the Psychosocial Wellbeing of Orphaned Children in Botswana," *African Journal of AIDS Research* 11, no. 3 (2012), 215–24.

7. Gerzon, Mark, *A Choice of Heroes: The Changing Face of American Manhood* (New York: Houghton Mifflin, 1982), 173–79.

8. Thanks to the input of Matthew Gutmann, Professor of Anthropology at Brown University.

9. http://www.bjs.gov/content/pub/pdf/tjvfox2.pdf.

10. http://www.washingtontimes.com/news/2012/dec/25/fathers-disappear-from-households-across-america/?page=all.

11. http://www.theguardian.com/lifeandstyle/2014/jun/28/mentoring-is-what-young-men-crave-band-of-brothers.

3. THE $3,000 PULLING SCHOOL

1. Thanks to Alex Mackintosh, Jo Scarratt, Nicholas Frend, Rachel Ramsey, RDF, and FYI for their fine work on "The Hunt for Real Men."

2. Stearns, Peter N., *Be a Man: Males in Modern Society* (New York: Holmes and Meier, 1990), 59.

3. Ibid., 60.

4. http://www.theguardian.com/world/2014/oct/30/libya-spiritual-leader-banned-uk-islamists.

5. https://www.independent.co.uk/news/uk/omar-bakri-muhammad-islamist-leader-seeks-return-to-uk-after-being-banned-in-wake-of-77-praise-9570963.html.

6. https://www.theguardian.com/world/2009/feb/12/far-right-dutch-mp-ban-islam.

7. http://www.nytimes.com/2015/03/19/world/europe/dieudonne-mbala-mbala-french-comedian-convicted-of-condoning-terrorism.html.

8. http://www.bbc.co.uk/news/uk-30119100.

4. YO! SUSHI DATING

1. https://outofthiscentury.wordpress.com/2010/02/13/nineteenth-century-courtship-advice/.

2. Harari, Yuval Noah, *Sapiens: A Brief History of Humankind* (London: Harvill Secker, 2014), 47.

3. http://freakonomics.com/2009/12/02/is-the-paradox-of-choice-not-so-paradoxical-after-all/.

4. https://www.ece.utah.edu/eceCTools/Probability/Combinatorics/ProbCombEx15.pdf.

5. https://ams.aaaa.org/eweb/upload/faqs/adexposures.pdf.

6. Epstein, Robert, Mayuri Pandit, and Mansi Thakar, *Journal of Comparative Family Studies* 44, no. 3 (May–June 2013).

7. Interview with Brian J. Willoughby, December 30, 2015.

8. Stearns, op. cit., 210.

9. Rotundo, E. Anthony, *American Manhood: Transformations in Masculinity from the Revolution to the Modern Era* (New York: Basic Books, 1993), 100.

10. Li, Norman P., et al., "Mate Preferences Do Predict Attraction and Choices in the Early Stages of Mate Selection," *Journal of Personality and Social Psychology* 105, no. 5 (2013): 757–76. http://ink.library.smu.edu.sg/soss_research/1396.

11. Diamond, Jared, *The Rise and Fall of the Third Chimpanzee* (New York: Vintage, 1991), 87.

12. Ibid., 84.

13. Stearns, op. cit., 59–60.

14. Ibid., 123.

15. Siedel Canby, Henry, *The Age of Confidence: Life in the Nineties* (New York: Farrar & Rinehart, 1934), 162.

16. http://www.nytimes.com/2015/02/15/nyregion/yale-restricts-a-fraternity-after-sexual-misconduct.html?_r=0.

17. Spiegelhalter, David, *Sex by Numbers: What Statistics Can Tell Us About Sexual Behaviour* (London: Profile Books, 2015), 27.

18. https://www.psychologytoday.com/us/blog/strictly-casual/201404/is-casual-sex-the-rise-in-america and https://ifstudies.org/blog/promiscuous-america-smart-secular-and-somewhat-less-happy.

19. Bethmann, Dirk, and Michael Kvasnicka, "World War II, Missing Men, and Out-of-Wedlock Childbearing," *Economic Journal* (March 2013).

20. Bailey, Beth L., *From Front Porch to Back Seat: Courtship in Twentieth-Century America* (Baltimore: Johns Hopkins University Press, 1989).

21. http://www.huffingtonpost.com/lauren-kay/why-nyc-women-should-consider-flying-across-the-country-to-find-men_b_4894602.html.

22. http://visualizing.nyc/nyc-zip-codes-singles-map/.

23. http://www.pewresearch.org/2009/10/15/the-states-of-marriage-and-divorce/.

24. https://www.washingtonpost.com/news/wonk/wp/2015/05/06/why-millennials-have-sex-with-fewer-partners-than-their-parents-did/?utm_term=.2d9efb279e07.

25. Spiegelhalter, op. cit., 30.

26. Diamond, op. cit., 66.

27. Ibid., 64.

28. https://www.cbsnews.com/news/changing-attitudes-about-premarital-sex-homosexuality/.

29. Bly, op. cit., 252–53.

30. Stearns, op. cit., 35–36.

31. Ibid., 126.

32. Kimmel, op. cit. (2005), 50.

33. Rotundo, op. cit., 120.

34. Collins, Marcus, *Modern Love: An Intimate History of Men and Women in Britain, 1900–2000* (New York: Atlantic Books, 2003), 208.

35. https://www.ted.com/talks/hannah_fry_the_mathematics_of_love /transcript?language=en.

36. Kimmel, op. cit. (2005), 131.

5. RELATIONSHIPS. OH MAN!

1. Ariely, Dan, and George Loewenstein, "The Heat of the Moment: The Effect of Sexual Arousal on Sexual Decision Making," *Journal of Behavioral Decision Making* 19 (2006).

2. Hibbert, Christopher, *The English, A Social History 1066–1945* (Paladin, 1988), 403–404.

3. Ibid., 405.

4. Bryson, Bill, *At Home: A Short History of Private Life* (illustrated edition) (New York: Doubleday, 2013), 131.

5. Diamond, op. cit., 80.

6. Spiegelhalter, op. cit., 43.

7. https://en.wikipedia.org/wiki/Academic_grading_in_the _United_States.

8. http://www.jewishencyclopedia.com/articles/10949-monogamy.

9. https://www.psychologytoday.com/blog/darwin-eternity/201109 /why-we-think-monogamy-is-normal.

10. Hibbert, op. cit., 400–401.

11. http://www.grreporter.info/en/world_wedding_industry_has _reached_amount_300_billion/11050.

12. http://www.ibisworld.com/industry/default.aspx?indid=2008.

13. A conservative estimate based on the US figure alone of $11 billion. http://www.nytimes.com/2013/05/05/fashion/weddings/how-americans -learned-to-love-diamonds.html?_r=1& and http://www.nytimes.com /2014/02/01/your-money/with-engagement-rings-love-meets-budget .html.

14. Based on the same logic and a figure of $12 billion in the US. See Kolpas, Norman and Katie Kolpas, *Practically Useless Information on Weddings* (Nashville: Thomas Nelson Publishers, 2005), 167.

15. Extrapolated from the US figure of $17 billion. http://www.busines-sinsider.com/valentines-day-gifts-and-spending-facts-2014-2?IR=T.

16. https://www.jonathanwstokes.com/blog/2015/04/18/are-romantic -comedies-profitable.

17. https://en.wikipedia.org/wiki/List_of_countries_by_GDP_ (PPP).

18. http://www.transparencymarketresearch.com/pressrelease/breakfast -cereals-industry.htm.

19. Diamond, op. cit., 59 and 81.

20. https://www.psychologytoday.com/blog/darwin-eternity/201109 /why-we-think-monogamy-is-normal.

21. Dixson, Alan F., *Primate Sexuality: Comparative Studies of the Prosimians, Monkeys, Apes, and Humans* (Oxford University Press, 2013), 299.

22. http://www.thestranger.com/seattle/SavageLove?oid=11412386.

23. Diamond, op. cit., 62.

24. Rubin, Roger, "Alternative Lifestyles Revisited, or Whatever Happened to Swingers, Group Marriages, and Communes?" *Journal of Family Issues* 22 (September 2001): 711–26.

25. Diamond, op. cit., 53.

26. Harari, op. cit., 42.

27. Diamond, op. cit., 18–19.

28. Harari, op. cit., 148.

29. Self, Will, *Great Apes* (London: Bloomsbury Publishing, 1997), xi–xii.

30. http://www.healthdata.org/news-release/nearly-one-third-world's-population-obese-or-overweight-new-data-show.

31. http://www.spiegel.de/international/world/sex-and-power-powerful-men-have-an-overactive-libido-a-765316.html.

32. http://www.imdb.com/title/tt0063135/quotes.

33. Diamond, op. cit., 63.

34. Arnold and Brady, op. cit., 417–18.

35. Ibid., 415–16.

36. Spiegelhalter, op. cit., 259–60.

37. https://www.psychologytoday.com/articles/201206/promise-promiscuity.

38. http://www.publications.parliament.uk/pa/ld199900/ldjudgmt/jd000727/smith-2.htm.

39. Collins, op. cit., 208.

40. http://lavistachurchofchrist.org/LVanswers/2013/01-28.html.

41. https://www.dailymail.co.uk/femail/article-1236435/Why-men-forgive-wifes-affair—theyd-expect-YOU-forgive-them.html.

42. https://www.fbi.gov/about-us/cjis/ucr/crime-in-the-u.s/2010/crime-in-the-u.s.-2010/tables/10shrtbl10.xls.

43. http://news.bbc.co.uk/1/hi/wales/south_east/8248942.stm.

44. http://news.bbc.co.uk/1/hi/health/4137506.stm.

45. http://www.jstor.org/stable/10.1086/504167?seq=1#page_scan_tab_contents.

46. Diamond, op. cit., 73.

47. https://www.theatlantic.com/daily-dish/archive/2010/04/whose-baby/188520.

48. Diamond, op. cit., 75–76.

49. http://www.bloomberg.com/news/articles/2013-07-02/cheating-wives-narrowed-infidelity-gap-over-two-decades.

50. https://www.relate.org.uk/sites/default/files/separation-divorce-fact-sheet-jan2014.pdf.

51. Spiegelhalter, op. cit., 41.

52. http://www.nytimes.com/2009/06/28/fashion/28marriage.html?pagewanted=all&_r=0.

53. http://www.economist.com/news/britain/21590905-new-study-points-curious-blend-attitudes-sex-love-cold-climate.

54. http://www.telegraph.co.uk/women/sex/10857870/The-closer-the-couple-the-better-the-sex-Not-so.html.

55. Hibbert, op. cit., 386.

56. http://www.washingtonpost.com/blogs/she-the-people/wp/2014/10/08/till-death-do-us-part-no-way-gray-divorce-on-the-rise/.

57. *Economist*, May 30, 2015, 21.

58. http://www.health.harvard.edu/newsletter_article/marriage-and-mens-health.

59. http://www.feelguide.com/2013/04/29/75-years-in-the-making-harvard-just-released-its-epic-study-on-what-men-require-to-live-a-happy-life/.

60. Stearns, op. cit., 76.

61. http://www.nytimes.com/2009/06/28/fashion/28marriage.html?pagewanted=all&_r=0.

62. Stearns, op. cit., 216.

63. http://www.economist.com/news/britain/21590905-new-study-points-curious-blend-attitudes-sex-love-cold-climate.

64. Harari, op. cit., 46.

65. http://www.qxmagazine.com/feature/continuing-our-series-looking-at-gay-shame-sexuality-this-week-simon-marks-trainee-dramatherapist-and-lgbt-activist/.

66. http://www.theatlantic.com/magazine/archive/2013/05/thanks-mom/309287/.

67. https://www.centreforsocialjustice.org.uk/core/wp-content/uploads/2016/08/CSJ-Press-Release-Lone-Parents.pdf.

68. https://slate.com/human-interest/2014/03/esther-perel-on-affairs-spouses-in-happy-marriages-cheat-and-americans-dont-understand-infidelity.html.

69. http://www.telegraph.co.uk/men/relationships/11025820/Can-an-open-marriage-ever-work-in-the-real-world.html.

70. http://www.pewresearch.org/fact-tank/2014/12/22/less-than-half-of-u-s-kids-today-live-in-a-traditional-family/.

71. de Botton, Alain, *Religion for Atheists: A Non-believer's Guide to the Uses of Religion* (London: Penguin, 2012), 63–66.

72. http://www.theatlantic.com/health/archive/2014/06/happily-ever-after/372573/.

73. Thanks to Charlotte de Botton for her wise thoughts on this.

74. http://www.reuters.com/article/2011/09/29/us-mexico-marriage-idUSTRE78S6TX20110929.

75. Hibbert, op. cit., 383.

76. Stearns, op. cit., 92.

77. Hibbert, op. cit., 390.

78. http://www.theatlantic.com/health/archive/2014/06/happily-ever-after/372573/.

79. http://news.bbc.co.uk/1/hi/sci/tech/3812483.stm.

7. A BAD DAY FOR A MELTDOWN

1. Soames, Mary, *Clementine Churchill* (New York: Doubleday, 2003).

2. https://www.thecalmzone.net/2014/02/onssuicidereport/.

3. http://www.cmha.ca/public_policy/men-and-mental-illness/.

4. http://www.bcmj.org/articles/silent-epidemic-male-suicide.

5. http://www.cmha.ca/public_policy/men-and-mental-illness/.

6. https://www.psychologytoday.com/us/blog/when-your-adult-child-breaks-your-heart/201504/women-and-mental-illness.

7. http://www.menshealthforum.org.uk/key-data-mental-health.

8. http://www.cmha.ca/public_policy/men-and-mental-illness/#. VJqmCr3YNQ.

9. https://www.statista.com/chart/11573/gender-of-inmates-in-us -federal-prisons-and-general-population/.

10. http://www.menshealthforum.org.uk/key-data-mental-health.

11. Rotundo, op. cit., 292.

12. http://www.mind.org.uk/media/273473/delivering-male.pdf, 2.

13. https://www.theguardian.com/society/2018/sep/04/fathers-men -get-posnatal-depression-too.

14. Reeves, A., M. McKee, and D. Stuckler, "Economic Suicides in the Great Recession in Europe and North America," *British Journal of Psychiatry* 205, no. 3 (September 2014): 246–47. DOI: 10.1192/bjp. bp.114.144766.

15. Office of National Statistics, UK.

16. http://www.mind.org.uk/media/273473/delivering-male.pdf, 26.

17. Rotundo, op. cit., 168.

18. Rotundo, op. cit., 186; and Kimmel, op. cit. (2005), 52.

19. Ibid.

20. Rotundo, op. cit., 187.

21. Kimmel, op. cit. (2005), 53.

22. Ibid., 52.

23. http://www.ncbi.nlm.nih.gov/pmc/articles/PMC3480686/ and Gerzon, op. cit., 224.

24. Harari, op. cit., 81.

25. https://eu.usatoday.com/story/news/nation/2014/05/12/mental-health -system-crisis/7746535/.

26. https://www.mentalhealthcommission.ca/sites/default/files/2016-06 /Investing_in_Mental_Health_FINAL_Version_ENG.pdf.

27. http://www.nimh.nih.gov/about/director/2011/the-global-cost-of
-mental-illness.shtml.

28. http://www.oecdbetterlifeindex.org/blog/the-cost-of-mental-illness
.htm.

29. http://www.theguardian.com/healthcare-network/2014/sep/02
/mental-health-low-priority-united-nations.

30. https://data.worldbank.org/indicator/NV.AGR.TOTL.
ZS?locations=US.

31. http://www.theguardian.com/sustainable-business/mental-health
-taboo-workplace-employers.

32. http://www.acas.org.uk/index.aspx?articleid=4337.

33. http://psychcentral.com/blog/archives/2013/10/02/need-help-for
-depression-try-acupuncture-instead-of-counseling/ and http://www
.scientificamerican.com/article/can-acupuncture-treat-depression/.

34. Harari, op. cit., 391.

8. HOW WAS YOUR DAY, DEAR?

1. https://www.thebalancecareers.com/what-is-the-average-hours
-per-week-worked-in-the-us-2060631.

2. http://www.bbc.co.uk/news/health-32069698.

3. James, Oliver, *Britain on the Couch: How Keeping up with the Joneses Has Depressed Us Since 1950* (London: Vermilion, 2010), 20.

4. Kimmel, Michael, *Angry White Men: American Masculinity at the End of an Era* (New York: Avalon, 2013), 180.

5. Pejtersen, J. H., H. Feveile, K. B. Christensen, and H. Burr, "Sickness Absence Associated with Shared and Open-Plan Offices—A National Cross-sectional Questionnaire Survey," *Scandinavian Journal of Work Environment and Health* 37, no. 5 (September 2011): 376–82. DOI: 10.5271/sjweh.3167.

6. http://www.newyorker.com/business/currency/the-open-office-trap.

7. Kimmel, op. cit. (2013), 45.

8. Stearns, op. cit., 163.

9. Harari, op. cit., 48–51.

10. Ibid., 49–50.

11. Stearns, op. cit., 23.

12. Kimmel, op. cit. (2005), 63.

13. Stearns, op. cit., 85.

14. http://cambriawillnotyield.blogspot.co.uk/2006/11/welsh-coal-miners -prayer.html.

15. http://www.theguardian.com/business/2001/dec/09/theobserver .observerbusiness14.

16. http://news.bbc.co.uk/1/hi/business/3549633.stm.

17. Stearns, op. cit., 97.

18. http://www.bls.gov/oes/current/oes339032.htm.

19. Bly, op. cit., ix.

20. *Economist,* May 30, 2015, 21.

21. Ibid., 19.

22. Kimmel, op. cit. (2013), 209 and https://www.stlouisfed.org/publications /regional-economist/october-2009/the-mancession-of-20082009 -its-big-but-its-not-great.

23. http://www.newyorker.com/business/currency/who-belongs-to-the -lower-middle-class-and-why-does-it-matter.

24. Kimmel, op. cit. (2013), 10–14.

25. *Economist,* May 30, 2015, 20.

26. http://www.mind.org.uk/news-campaigns/news/stressed-out-staff -feel-unsupported-at-work-says-mind.

27. Ibid.

28. https://www.telegraph.co.uk/business/0/female-bosses-ftse-100/.

29. *The Why Factor,* BBC World Service, May 22, 2015.

30. http://www.forbes.com/sites/lesliebradshaw/2011/11/08/why -luck-has-nothing-to-do-with-it/.

31. http://www.medicaldaily.com/how-stress-divides-sexes -why-do-men-withdraw-while-women-become-more-social-271488.

32. https://www.theguardian.com/commentisfree/2018/oct/06 /homophobic-mismogynist-racist-brazil-jair-bolsonaro.

33. http://www.pewresearch.org/2009/02/03/limbaugh-holds-onto -his-niche-conservative-men/.

34. Kimmel, op. cit. (2013), 109.

35. Ibid., 201.

36. Ibid., 73.

37. http://www.huffingtonpost.com/michael-kimmel/the-unbearable -whiteness_2_b_2350931.html and http://www.huffingtonpost.com/tio -hardiman/unemployment-and-violence_b_4751144.html.

38. https://home.chicagopolice.org/wp-content/uploads/2019/03 /Chicago-Police-Department-Annual-Report-2017.pdf.

39. http://www.pewresearch.org/fact-tank/2013/08/21/through-good-times -and-bad-black-unemployment-is-consistently-double-that-of -whites/.

40. http://www.theguardian.com/society/2014/jan/08/minority -ethnic-workers-more-often-unemployed.

41. National Health Service, *Mental Health: National Service Frameworks* (London: NHS, 1999), 77.

42. http://www.prisonreformtrust.org.uk/projectsresearch/race.

43. http://www.usnews.com/news/articles/2013/06/12/gun-owners-still -overwhelmingly-white-males.

44. *Economist,* May, 30, 2015, 20, quoting from Hanna Rosin's *The End of Men.*

45. http://www.telegraph.co.uk/women/womens-business/11307493 /Gender-pay-gap-closes-as-more-women-join-higher-rate-taxpayer -club.html.

46. https://www.theatlantic.com/education/archive/2017/08/why-men-are-the-new-college-minority/536103/.

47. http://www.pewresearch.org/fact-tank/2018/04/09/gender-pay-gap-facts/.

48. http://www.theatlantic.com/business/archive/2013/09/the-overhyped-rise-of-stay-at-home-dads/279279/.

49. Harari, op. cit., 393–94.

50. Kimmel, op. cit. (2005), 29.

51. Ibid., 31.

52. Ibid., 32.

53. https://www.theguardian.com/tv-and-radio/2015/jul/02/the-island-bear-grylls-135000-applicants-channel-4.

9. SET OUR TESTOSTERONE FREE

1. Kimmel, op. cit. (2013), 221.

2. Stearns, op. cit., 86.

3. Nye, Robert A., *Masculinity and Male Codes of Honor in Modern France* (Oxford University Press, 1993), 185.

4. Ibid., 201 and 211.

5. Ibid., 177.

6. Ibid., 216.

7. http://www.usnews.com/news/articles/2015/03/06/gang-violence-is-on-the-rise-even-as-overall-violence-declines.

8. https://www.cdc.gov/violenceprevention/pdf/NISVS-infographic-2016.pdf.

9. http://www.independent.co.uk/news/uk/crime/record-numbers-of-women-held-for-violent-crimes-1882111.html and http://aic.gov.au/publications/current%20series/rip/21-40/rip29.html.

10. https://www.theguardian.com/society/2010/sep/05/men-victims -domestic-violence.

11. Kimmel, op. cit. (2005), 77.

12. https://history.msu.edu/hst324/files/2013/05/muscular.pdf.

13. Ibid.

14. Rotundo, op. cit., 226.

15. Kenway, Jane, Anna Kraack, and Anna Hickey-Moody, *Masculinity Beyond the Metropolis* (New York: Palgrave Macmillan, 2006), 178.

16. Trimpop, R. M., *The Psychology of Risk Taking Behavior* (Amsterdam: North-Holland Publishing, 1994), 219.

17. http://bigthink.com/videos/why-men-drive-fast-and-take-chances.

18. https://www.apa.org/monitor/julaug06/frisky.

19. http://bigthink.com/videos/why-men-drive-fast-and-take-chances.

20. https://www.psychologytoday.com/articles/200011/are-you -risk-taker.

21. Bly, op. cit., p. 182.

22. http://www.nydailynews.com/news/national/boy-7-suspended-throwing -imaginary-grenade-article-1.1256200.

23. http://www.cbsnews.com/news/examiner-recommends-school -board-uphold-pop-tart-suspension/.

24. http://www.manchestereveningnews.co.uk/news/altrincham -grammar-school-boys-pupil-7174142.

25. https://www.telegraph.co.uk/sport/othersports/schoolsports/11092344 /Is-it-game-over-for-school-playing-fields.html.

26. http://www.theguardian.com/world/2014/jan/08/research-american -children-exercise-obesity-health.

27. https://www.nationaltrust.org.uk/document-1355766991839/.

28. Ibid.

29. Stearns, op. cit., 114.

30. http://www.medicalnewstoday.com/articles/279281.php.

31. Winn, William E., "Tom Brown's Schooldays and the Development of 'Muscular Christianity,'" *Church History* (Cambridge University Press, March 1960), vol. 29, no. 1, 64–73. http://www.jstor.org/stable/3161617.

32. Rotundo, op. cit., 295.

33. Kimmel, op. cit. (2005), 65.

34. https://www.nationalchurchillmuseum.org/churchill-in-world-war-i-and-aftermath.html.

35. https://winstonchurchill.org/publications/churchill-bulletin/bulletin-057-mar-2013/winston-churchill-for-traders-a-analysts.

36. Broyles, Jr., William, "Why Men Love War," *Brothers in Arms* (New York: Knopf, 1986).

37. Gerzon, op. cit., 32.

38. Ibid., 53.

39. http://www.theguardian.com/film/2014/jul/17/why-so-obsessed-second-world-war-films.

40. http://www.independent.co.uk/news/uk/politics/we-need-more-wars-head-of-controversial-private-outsourcing-firm-blames-lack-of-conflict-for-spectacular-collapse-in-army-recruitment-since-it-took-charge-8952799.html.

41. http://edition.cnn.com/2015/02/10/politics/isis-foreign-fighters-combat; https://www.npr.org/sections/parallels/2018/02/05/583407221/americans-in-isis-some-300-tried-to-join-12-have-returned-to-u-s?t=1548350727921; and https://www.washingtonpost.com/graphics/2018/world/isis-returning-fighters/?noredirect=on&utm_term=.94aa95b2e7de.

42. https://www.nytimes.com/2018/09/21/us/army-recruiting-shortage.html.

43. http://www.theatlantic.com/international/archive/2015/03/isis-and-the-foreign-fighter-problem/387166/.

44. Ibid.

45. http://www.telegraph.co.uk/news/uknews/terrorism-in-the-uk/11274764/Man-who-joined-Syrian-terrorist-training-camp-after-row-with-wife-is-jailed.html.

46. http://blogs.reuters.com/great-debate/2014/10/16/joining-islamic-state-is-about-sex-and-aggression-not-religion/.

47. http://www.npr.org/2015/06/21/416167159/for-a-british-man-fighting-isis-was-simply-the-right-thing-to-do.

48. http://www.independent.co.uk/news/world/middle-east/macer-gifford-british-man-joins-kurds-to-fight-isis-in-syria-10034768.html.

49. https://www.theguardian.com/world/2015/jun/11/macer-gifford-briton-fight-isis-shine-light-conflict.

50. https://www.rand.org/pubs/research_reports/RR1928.html?adbsc=social_20180320_2212921&adbid=975928167633334272&adbpl=tw&adbpr=22545453.

51. https://www.ptsd.va.gov/understand/common/common_veterans.asp.

52. https://www.smithsonianmag.com/science-nature/over-quarter-million-vietnam-war-veterans-still-have-ptsd-180955997/.

53. http://www.bbc.co.uk/news/uk-23259865 and http://www.abc.net.au/news/2014-04-22/number-of-soldiers-committing-suicide-triples-afghan-combat-toll/5403122.

54. http://www.theguardian.com/world/2013/feb/01/us-military-suicide-epidemic-veteran.

55. https://www.va.gov/opa/pressrel/pressrelease.cfm?id=4074.

56. Thanks to the brilliant work of Liam McArdle, Janet Lee, and *The Culture Show* team on making *Art for Heroes*.

57. Gerzon, op. cit., 36.

58. https://www.bbc.co.uk/news/magazine-27067615.

59. Nye, op. cit., 217–18.

60. Based on the tenuous listings of Swiss films on Wikipedia—not the most concrete stat in this book! https://en.wikipedia.org/wiki/Category:Swiss_films.

61. Gerzon, op. cit., 33.

62. http://www.eurekalert.org/pub_releases/2012-07/uoc-rtf071312.php.

63. http://www.spiegel.de/international/germany/the-twilight-of-the-civvies-germany-to-scale-back-mandatory-civilian-service-a-692751.html.

64. http://www.jrf.org.uk/publications/poverty-and-wealth-across-britain-1968-2005.

65. Thanks to the genius of Will Daws, Kate Townsend, Simon Brown, Fiona Cleary, Danny Collins, Jonathan Bell, and Sam Anstiss on *The Great Granny Chart Invasion*.

66. Caputo, Philip, *A Rumor of War* (London: Pimlico, 1977), xvii.

67. Broyles, op. cit.

68. *Science,* June 11, 2010, 1325. DOI: 10.1126/science.328.5984.1325-c.

69. Stearns, op. cit., 4.

70. Hibbert, op. cit., 375.

71. Kimmel, op. cit. (2013), 50.

72. Rotundo, op. cit., 143.

73. BBC oral history project, http://www.bbc.co.uk/programmes/p00n4j54.

74. https://aboutaberdeen.com/The-Grill-Bar-Oldest-Aberdeen-Pub-Union-Street.

75. http://www.iea.org.uk/sites/default/files/publications/files/Briefing_Closing%20time_web.pdf.

76. https://www.bostonglobe.com/lifestyle/style/2016/02/17/what-killing-boston-dive-bars/ooEgqyF3LqnPQpCIadnKRL/story.html.

77. http://www.economist.com/news/christmas-specials/21636688-though-thriving-parts-asia-golf-struggling-america-and-much-europe.

78. Kimmel, op. cit. (2013), 115.
79. https://pdfs.semanticscholar.org/4561/e35b5765f3eea29503b7cb-77dec5e3fe9b65.pdf.
80. Ibid.

10. SPARE PART ON A PORN SET

1. Thanks to Alex Mackintosh, Seth Goolnik, Sally Hewitt, Tom Fulford, Danny Collins, Sam Anstiss, Will Daws, Stuart Cabb, and Plum Pictures for great stuff on *Hardcore Profits*.
2. Spiegelhalter, op. cit., 108, quoting from historian Alan Hunt.
3. Hibbert, op. cit., 406 and http://theappendix.net/posts/2013/06/this-misterie-of-fucking-a-sex-manual-from-1680.
4. http://youporn.com.hypestat.com.
5. http://www.extremetech.com/computing/123929-just-how-big-are-porn-sites/2.
6. http://www.alexa.com/siteinfo/youporn.com.
7. http://www.huffingtonpost.com/2013/05/03/internet-porn-stats_n_3187682.html.
8. Gunelius, Susan, *Building Brand Value the Playboy Way* (New York: Palgrave Macmillan, 2009), 77–78.
9. https://bellisario.psu.edu/assets/pdf/pennsylvania-center-for-the-first-amendment/vanderbilt09.pdf.
10. Arnold and Brady, op. cit., 211.
11. Spiegelhalter, op. cit., 244.
12. http://www.theatlantic.com/politics/archive/2014/03/most-people-think-watching-porn-is-morally-wrong/284240/.
13. http://www.theguardian.com/law/2015/mar/17/three-judges-removed-and-a-fourth-resigns-for-viewing-pornography-at-work.

14. There are interesting thoughts and cases on this question at: http://barristerblogger.com/2015/03/18/were-the-three-porn-viewing-judges-rightly-sacked/.

15. http://www.independent.co.uk/voices/a-chief-justice-got-away-with-murder-1169087.html.

16. *Nature Neuroscience,* 7 (2004): 411–16. Published online 7 March 2004; DOI: 10.1038/nn1208. https://www.nature.com/articles/nn1208.

17. https://www.psychologytoday.com/blog/sex-dawn/201004/why-do-breasts-mesmerize.

18. Spiegelhalter, op. cit., 65.

19. Ibid., 246, quoting analysis by Jon Millward.

20. Brundage, James A., "Let Me Count the Ways: Canonists and Theologians Contemplate Coital Positions," *Journal of Medieval History* 10, no. 2 (June 1984): 81–93.

21. http://news.bbc.co.uk/1/hi/uk/7180401.stm.

22. https://www.psychologytoday.com/blog/inside-porn-addiction/201112/is-porn-really-destroying-500000-marriages-annually.

23. Spiegelhalter, op. cit., 247–48.

24. http://www.bbc.co.uk/news/education-32115162.

25. http://www.bbc.co.uk/newsbeat/article/32916056/porn-addiction-i-couldnt-focus-on-everyday-activities.

26. *Journal of the American Medical Association Pediatrics* 168, no. 1 (2014): 34–39. DOI: 10.1001/jamapediatrics.2013.2915.

27. http://www.theguardian.com/culture/2015/mar/16/pornography-belongs-classroom-professor-denmark.

11. A JEALOUS ATHEIST

1. Harari, op. cit., 54 and 212–18.

2. Greenstone, Gerry, 'The History of Bloodletting," *BC Medical Journal* 52, no. 1 (January/February 2010).

3. http://www.history.com/news/a-brief-history-of-bloodletting.

4. http://www.pewresearch.org/fact-tank/2015/05/06/5-facts -about-prayer/.

5. https://www.psychologytoday.com/blog/the-secular-life/201409/ why-are-women-more-religious-men.

6. The theory of Professor Rodney Stark, http://www.washington.edu /news/2002/12/18/why-are-men-less-religious-it-may-be-form-of -risk-taking-impulsivity-just-as-criminal-behavior-is/.

7. http://www.huffingtonpost.com/richard-dawkins/why-there -almost-certainl_b_32164.html.

8. http://www.huffingtonpost.com/2011/01/15/british-study-links -sprea_n_809394.html.

9. Koenig, Harold G., "Research on Religion, Spirituality, and Mental Health: A Review," *Canadian Journal of Psychiatry* (2008).

10. Collinge, William J., *Historical Dictionary of Catholicism* (Scarecrow Press, 2012), 102.

11. http://www.provenmen.org/2014pornsurvey/pornography-use-and -addiction/.

12. de Botton, op. cit., 71.

13. Ibid., 294.

14. https://www.psychologytoday.com/blog/why-we-worry/201206 /the-psychological-effects-tv-news.

15. Shermer, Michael, *The Believing Brain: From Spiritual Faiths to Political Convictions: How We Construct Beliefs and Reinforce Them as Truths* (London: Hachette UK, 2012), 198–201 and https://www .newscientist.com/article/dn7147-genes-contribute-to-religious - inclination/.

16. Bukowski, Charles, *Women* (London: Virgin Books, 2009), 260.

17. http://www.tabletmag.com/jewish-life-and-religion/162315/aphrodisiacs-valentines-day.

18. Bly, op. cit., 252–53.

12. PATERNITY TEST

1. Howe, Tasha R., *Marriages and Families in the 21st Century: A Bioecological Approach* (Hoboken, NJ: John Wiley & Sons, 2011), 283.

2. Kroeger, Mary, *Impact of Birthing Practices on Breastfeeding: Protecting the Mother and Baby Continuum* (Burlington, MA: Jones & Bartlett Learning, 2004), 53.

3. Kimmel, op. cit. (2013), 140.

4. http://www.telegraph.co.uk/news/health/news/9668962/Fathers-to-be-to-join-partners-in-birthing-pools.html.

5. http://www.catholicnewsagency.com/news/a-society-without-fathers-is-a-society-of-orphans-pope-francis-says-55843/.

6. Based on a French study: Rolland, M., et al., "Decline in Semen Concentration and Morphology in a Sample of 26,609 Men Close to General Population between 1989 and 2005 in France," *Human Reproduction* (December 4, 2012), 462–70.

7. Carlsen, E., et al., "Evidence for Decreasing Quality of Semen during Past 50 Years," *BMJ* 305 (1992): 609.

8. http://www.ewg.org/research/propyl-paraben.

9. Martinez, J. and J. E. Lewi, "An Unusual Case of Gynecomastia Associated with Soy Product Consumption," *Endocrine Practice* 14, no. 4 (May–June 2008):415–18.

10. Kim, Pilyoung, and James E. Swain, "Sad Dads: Paternal Post-partum Depression," *Psychiatry* 4, no. 2 (Edgmont, February 2007): 35–47.

11. Stearns, op. cit., 130.

12. Cleves, Rachel Hope, "Wayland, Francis (1796–1865)," in Fass, Paula S., ed., *Encyclopedia of Children and Childhood in History and Society* (New York: Macmillan, 2004).

13. Arnold and Brady, op. cit., 105–106.

14. Hibbert, op. cit., 393.

15. Stearns, op. cit., 58.

16. Arnold and Brady, op. cit., 171.

17. Stearns, op. cit., 206–207.

18. Ibid., 172.

19. Kimmel, op. cit. (2013), 142.

20. http://www.theguardian.com/lifeandstyle/2014/jun/15/fathers-spend-more-time-with-children-than-in-1970s.

21. http://www.cdc.gov/nchs/data/nhsr/nhsr071.pdf.

22. http://www.pewresearch.org/fact-tank/2015/06/18/5-facts-about-todays-fathers/.

23. https://www.cdc.gov/nchs/data/nhsr/nhsr071.pdf.

24. http://www.pewsocialtrends.org/2013/03/14/modern-parenthood-roles-of-moms-and-dads-converge-as-they-balance-work-and-family/.

25. http://www.hmc.org.uk/wp-content/uploads/2013/11/Insight_issue_4_Summer2015_2.pdf.

26. Hibbert, op. cit., 392.

27. https://www.thelocal.se/20120611/41358.

28. https://sweden.se/quickfact/parental-leave/.

29. http://www.pewsocialtrends.org/2014/06/05/growing-number-of-dads-home-with-the-kids/.

30. http://sowf.men-care.org.

31. *Economist,* May 30, 2015, 21.

32. http://www.pewsocialtrends.org/2009/10/01/the-harried-life-of-the-working-mother/.

33. http://www.economist.com/news/united-states/21600998-after-falling-years-proportion-mums-who-stay-home-rising-return.

34. Kimmel, op. cit. (2013), 142.

35. *New Yorker,* February 12, 2007.

36. Psychologist Dr. Michael Thompson, coauthor of *Raising Cain,* talking on *Men's Hour,* July 31, 2011.

37. http://www.economist.com/blogs/economist-explains/2014/07/economist-explains-15.

38. http://sowf.s3.amazonaws.com/wp-content/uploads/2015/06/08181421/State-of-the-Worlds-Fathers_23June2015.pdf.

39. Ferrarini, T., and T. Norström, "Family Policy, Economic Development, and Infant Mortality: A Longitudinal Comparative Analysis." *International Journal of Social Welfare* 19 (2010): S89–S102.

40. http://www.ilo.org/wcmsp5/groups/public/---dgreports/---dcomm/---publ/documents/publication/wcms_242615.pdf.

41. https://www.theguardian.com/lifeandstyle/2013/nov/02/men-single-dad-father-surrogacy-adoption.

42. http://www.nytimes.com/2013/02/24/business/fathers-seek-advertising-that-does-not-ridicule.html?_r=0.

43. http://phys.org/news/2006-11-men-main-gender-wars.html.

44. http://www.her.ie/life/missing-milestones-survey-shows-many-fathers-are-missing-out-on-important-days-because-of-work-pressures/145710.

45. http://sowf.s3.amazonaws.com/wp-content/uploads/2015/06/08181421/State-of-the-Worlds-Fathers_23June2015.pdf.

46. Kraemer, S., "The Fragile Male," *BMJ* 321 (2000): 1609–12; Ferrarini, T., and T. Norström, "Family Policy, Economic Development, and Infant Mortality: A Longitudinal Comparative Analysis," *International Journal of Social Welfare* 19 (2010): S89–S102.

47. http://www.pewsocialtrends.org/2011/06/15/a-tale-of-two-fathers and http://www.natcen.ac.uk/news-media/press-releases/2013/november/nine-in-ten-fathers-say-they-keep-in-touch-with-non-resident-children/.

48. https://www.centreforsocialjustice.org.uk/library/fractured-families-stability-matters.

49. Ratzinger, Joseph (Pope Benedict XVI), *The God of Jesus Christ: Meditations on the Triune God* (San Francisco: Ignatius Press, 2008), 29.

50. https://raywilliams.ca/the-decline-of-fatherhood-and-male-identity-crisis.

51. Kimmel, op. cit. (2013), 151.

52. http://www.pewsocialtrends.org/2011/06/15/a-tale-of-two-fathers/.

53. http://www.telegraph.co.uk/men/relationships/fatherhood/11647915/Are-divorced-dads-really-treated-fairly-by-the-family-courts.html.

54. Berman at Oxford University sociology department, divorce conference 2013.

55. http://www.theatlantic.com/magazine/archive/2000/05/the-war-against-boys/304659/.

56. Center on Education Policy.

57. https://www.government.se/legal-documents/2010/07/sou-201053/.

58. http://jama.jamanetwork.com/article.aspx?articleid=1832542#joi140013t3.

59. http://www.telegraph.co.uk/news/health/news/10978836/Number-of-women-travelling-to-America-to-choose-sex-of-child-rises-20.html.

60. https://poseidon01.ssrn.com/delivery.php?ID=519021121111026081018088085092006026004062027018026066117023102007113119075090072067043099051062060010113071003083028091105122039071017081004074103075101119014088024060040103027071090125018083028118013069000009022118079123025030071099003106109069090&EXT=pdf.

61. http://msan.wceruw.org/conferences/2013-miniConf/J-Nov2013%20breakout%20ppt.pdf.

62. Stearns, op. cit., 78.

63. http://darkwing.uoregon.edu/~adoption/archive/SpenceRPT.htm.

64. Kimmel, op. cit. (2005), 97.

65. http://www.economist.com/news/international/21645759-boys-are
-being-outclassed-girls-both-school-and-university-and-gap.

66. Ruspini, E. et al., eds., *Men and Masculinities around the World:
Transforming Men's Practices* (New York: Palgrave Macmillan, 2011),
163–64.

67. Speaking on *Men's Hour*, July 31, 2011.

68. http://www.edu.gov.on.ca/eng/curriculum/meread_andhow.pdf.

69. http://www.theatlantic.com/sexes/archive/2013/06/stop-penalizing
-boys-for-not-being-able-to-sit-still-at-school/276976/ and http://therite
journey.com/assets/Independence-Magazine-The-Rite-Journey1.pdf.

70. http://people.terry.uga.edu/cornwl/research/cmvp.genderdiffs.pdf.

71. https://www.nationaltrust.org.uk/document-1355766991839/.

72. Blyton, Enid, *Five Fall into Adventure* (Hodder, reissued 1997).

73. http://www.birminghampost.co.uk/news/local-news/police-arrest
-detain-three-children-3981499.

74. Adams, J., "Risk and Morality: Three Framing Devices," in Ericson,
R. V., and A. Doyle, eds., *Risk and Morality* (University of Toronto
Press, 2003).

75. http://www.theguardian.com/education/2008/aug/03/schools.
children.

76. Faber Taylor, A., et al., "Coping with ADD: The Surprising Connection
to Green Play Settings," *Environment and Behaviour* 33 (Jan 2001):
54–77, quoted in National Trust report.

77. http://bmjopen.bmj.com/content/3/5/e002646.full.pdf+html?
sid=81b1351b-1ad6-4fca-a2e7-eaa7cbf951be and https://www.cdc.
gov/mmwr/volumes/67/wr/mm6750a1.htm.

78. http://www.thesundaytimes.co.uk/sto/news/uk_news/Education
/article1461987.ece.

79. http://www.economist.com/news/international/21645759-boys-are
    -being-outclassed-girls-both-school-and-university-and-gap.
80. http://www.telegraph.co.uk/news/uknews/5934226/Hunter-
    gatherer-brains-make-men-and-women-see-things-differently.html.
81. Bly, op. cit., 199.
82. http://www.washingtonpost.com/sf/national/2015/05/16/a-fathers
    -initiative/ and https://www.nytimes.com/2008/06/16/us/politics/15cnd
    -obama.html.
83. Stearns, op. cit., 19.

13. CONCLUSION: RECLAIM THE SPEAR

1. http://www.theguardian.com/world/2011/may/15/arab-spring-tunisia
   -the-slap;   http://www.nytimes.com/2011/01/22/world/africa/22sidi
   .html?_r=0;   http://www.theguardian.com/world/2011/jan/20/tunisian
   -fruit-seller-mohammed-bouazizi;   http://www.spiegel.de/international
   /world/the-fruits-of-mohamed-the-small-tunisian-town-that
   -sparked-the-arab-revolution-a-751278.html; and http://www.worldaffairs
   journal.org/blog/michael-j-totten/woman-who-blew-arab-world.
2. http://time.com/16378/sigma-alpha-epsilon-frat-bans-initiations/.
3. *Economist,* May 30, 2015, 20.
4. http://www.bjs.gov/content/pub/pdf/pim09st.pdf.
5. http://www.upi.com/blog/2013/10/21/Report-Men-need-to-see
   -their-friends-twice-a-week-for-health-reasons/5341382374912/.

ABOUT THE AUTHOR

Tim Samuels is an award-winning documentary filmmaker, broadcaster, and journalist.

Tim has been a leading name on the BBC for many years. He now also appears as a global correspondent on the National Geographic channel.

Tim's films have won the top UK and international honors, including best documentary at the World Television Festival and three Royal Television Society Awards. He has written for the *New York Times*, the *Guardian*, and *GQ*. Tim's acclaimed new podcast, *All Hail Kale*, was the number one new BBC podcast according to the London *Evening Standard*.

Future Man, when published in Britain—as *Who Stole My Spear?*—was an Amazon bestseller.

Born in Manchester, England, Tim now lives in London but works between the UK and US. Visit Tim's site at www.tim-samuels.com.